A Wallflower
No More

BUILDING A NEW LIFE AFTER
EMOTIONAL AND SEXUAL ABUSE

JAYNE MAAS FREEMAN

Jayne Freeman

Freeman, Jayne Maas.
A wallflower no more : building a new life after emotional and sexual abuse / Jayne Maas Freeman.
    p. cm.
Summary: "A resource for survivors of emotional and sexual abuse that offers practical steps to self-mastery and healing"--Provided by publisher.
Includes bibliographical references.
ISBN 0-9762224-3-4 (alk. paper)
1. Adult child sexual abuse victims--Sexual behavior. 2. Adult child sexual abuse victims--Rehabilitation. 3. Hygiene, Sexual. 4. Sexually transmitted diseases--Psychological aspects. I. Title.

RC569.5.A28F746 2005
362.76'4--dc22
                                    2005010450

For interviews or to schedule workshops, contact:
The Hired Pen
877-277-6649

Published by Acacia Publishing, Inc.
1366 East Thomas Road, Suite 305
Phoenix, Arizona 85014
www.acaciapublishing.com
Printed and bound in Canada.

Table of Contents

Dedication

With a humble heart, grateful spirit, undying courage and love, I dedicate this book to the brave women and men who are in a daily struggle just to survive. You are the ones who don't want a handout, but a hand up. You find yourself in daily crisis with no way out of the situations you're in. They may not be of your own making, but nonetheless you are there anyway!

Secretly you dream of what seems to be the impossible dream of a better life for you and your children. However, exhaustion takes its toll by the end of the day's struggle. You fall asleep wondering if you'll even make it through tomorrow, much less ever achieve anything more.

A Wallflower No More is a practical guide to self-empowerment to help get you where you want to be. Make no mistake about it: if I can do it so can you.

To my four sons: guys, you are the reason I had to break the cycle of abuse in our family. You gave me the strength to make it through it all.

Foreword

Over a 10-year period from 1985–1995, I had the opportunity to be involved in a therapy group for adult women who were abused as children. I initially arranged the group and asked two female therapists to facilitate it. At the last minute, one of the leaders could not participate and the other asked me to sit in on the first group to support her. As a male therapist, I was reluctant to sit in on an all-female therapy group. However, the apprehension turned out to be in my head as I was readily accepted in the group. Six months into the group, the other female therapist changed jobs and I found myself facilitating the group alone for the next nine years. The group of eight to 14 women met once a week on Tuesday mornings. The scheduled three-hour group always ran overtime and five- to six-hour sessions were typical.

It was clear to me from the start that the 250–300 women who attended the group over the years needed someone to hear their story. Many also needed a *male* to listen to their story. I often symbolized the husbands, boyfriends, grandfathers, brothers, uncles, teachers, bosses, ministers, and police officers who had used and abused these women. Many times, I could see in the eyes of the woman speaking that she saw her abuser's face rather than mine. It was the most intense psychotherapy I have been a part of in my 32-year career.

Although there were many consistent themes to the stories of the women who bravely told of their abuse, every story was unique both in the level of betrayal and in the personal suffering that was always solitary.

I learned a great deal from these brave women. I learned about what happened in the shadows of well-to-do families where fathers were pillars of the community or of the church during the day, and sinister purveyors of terror at night. I learned about the thought patterns that develop when a child is used as a pawn for sick amusement or as a source of perverted gratification.

I also learned how the women tried to cope and make it through another day, even decades after the abuse had stopped. But for these and thousands of other abuse survivors, in their minds, the abuse never did stop. Some of the women had better coping styles than others, and some never found a way to cope—two group members committed suicide during the 10 years.

Jayne Freeman was not a member of this group, but she could have been. In reading *A Wallflower No More*, I was transported in my mind back to the thousands of hours of hearing the stories of abuse, betrayal, and heroic efforts to keep going each day. Although Jayne's personal story presented in these pages would not be unusual in our group, the resilience she has displayed time and time again would certainly place her among the extraordinary women who did not stop with coping, but prevailed against all odds.

While *A Wallflower No More* may be in some respects every traumatized woman's story of pain and betrayal, Jayne's response to her unsupportive world is unusual and exceptional. Because it is so extraordinary, this story is worth sharing with many other traumatized individuals.

Jayne's story is one of courage, endurance, and persistence that must come in part from a spiritual wellspring deep in her soul. Life is difficult enough without people who are supposed to provide love and support betraying you at every turn. How did she manage to not only keep going but to keep her dreams alive along the way? While the suggestions in the second half of the book can be immensely helpful, something deep within Jayne told her at each moment in her life that something much better was possible and even available.

Child abuse and sexual abuse in particular have now come out of the closet in our culture. We now know that the number one medical problem in the United States among children is being physically, emotionally and mentally abused by parents or family members. We also know that as many as one out of every four children, males and females, is subjected to some form of sexual betrayal growing up. The stories of secrecy and pain are in our newspapers, our movies and on the nightly news. Jayne's personal story no longer surprises us because we have heard similar stories many times before. But Jayne's fight to hold onto her dreams and possibilities is unusual indeed and bears scrutiny and reflection. While fundamentally a story of overcoming childhood abuse, Jayne's story is one of resilience in the face of overwhelming odds and becoming the author of her own story, and the director of her own play.

As low as abuse and betrayal take us in *A Wallflower No More*, beating the odds and prevailing in the search for self take us as high as the human condition can soar. Jayne did not lose her hope, and she did not lose her faith in her Heavenly Father. Perhaps the fact that Jayne is a real person who really went through all the things and did all the things in this book provides a degree of hope for all abused people everywhere. Her story and her life are profound not because of what went wrong, but because of what went right. The strength of the human spirit, while supported and guided by the divine spirit, is a force that can overcome torture, concentration camps, terror and abuse. The beauty of the self, forged in fire, is all the more beautiful due to the heat of the furnace it has gone through.

It is unfortunate that Jayne's story is so painful and difficult. It is also unfortunate that Jayne's reliance is not the story of every abused child, teen and adult—but it could be. When regular people do extraordinary things, they give hope to all the rest of us. Read these pages carefully, consider the suggestions thoughtfully, and then turn your attention to your own story. Consider your life goals and dreams and then start your own journey to "Get it done!"

Dave Ziegler, Ph.D.

Acknowledgments

On March 4, 2004, after seven years of pregnancy and 40 hours of intense labor, *A Wallflower No More* was birthed in Stockton, California!

Although a labor of love, during the seven years it took to write this manuscript, I dealt with a great deal of apprehension. Twelve years ago, the idea for the book came to me. For the first three years, I brushed it off because I was in intense recovery trying to deal with all that life was handing me at the time.

When the reality hit me that it wasn't my idea but Our Heavenly Father's, I started writing stories of my life with His encouragement but no idea where it was all going. A reality came to me that the subject matter was extremely intense, to say the least. My family and friends were already thinking I was strange because of my questions and demands of them. All the while I was trying to grasp the magnitude of what had happened to me in childhood. Putting it into words just flat-out scared me.

For the next three years, Our Heavenly Father and I would have an ongoing conversation about "the book." I feared for my earthly life, but he told me many others were waiting for the book to help them. He would protect and guide me.

I feared what my family would say, especially my mother. I expressed my concern for her once I wrote the book. She quieted those fears by saying, "If one woman or one child can be spared a life of hell by you telling our story, then do it." What courage it took her to say that!

I feared that the man I had fallen in love with wouldn't want a woman with my past, much less one who would tell the world about her childhood terror. If it weren't for his encouragement, calm support, and unconditional love, *A Wallflower No More* would have remained in my computer forever. **Bob Freeman, I Love You, Sweetheart!**

Also, special thanks to two awesome women, Aurora Ashton and Michelle LaVigueur, authors of the poems in *A Wall Flower No More*.

Aurora honored my literary efforts by writing "A Gentle Thunder." She has struggled for years to successfully overcome a childhood trauma. You go, girl!

While going through a terrifying phase in her life, raising her son and working on her bachelor's degree, Michelle wrote "Ripping at my Heart." With Our Heavenly Father beside you, no one can stop you.

These women, and many others I have known through the years, remind me daily why *A Wallflower No More* had to be written. Thank you, for your love and encouragement all these years.

Don, Joan and Cindy — three angels disguised as masters of the written word.

And to Terry, the greatest mentor alive, thanks for everything!

There were others, too many to list, but you know who you are. You can be assured you touched my life! When I needed the encouragement, love and support, you were there. We are all in this life together. I believe that 'things' don't just happen, they happen for a reason. Thank you from the bottom of my heart and the depths of my soul.

Jayne

x

"And whosoever shall offend one of these little ones

that believe in me, it is better for him that a

millstone were hanged about his neck, and he were

cast into the sea."

Mark 9:42

There are no words that can express

my deep feelings of gratitude and love toward

Our Heavenly Father.

Childhood

Childhood

The blissful ignorance of childhood came to a crashing halt for me when I was just six years old. As I lay warm and snug under a mountain of blankets on the living room floor, I was surprised to feel Max on top of me, putting his hands all over me. He was taking off my pajamas with one hand, while covering my mouth with the other; I tried to get out from under him, but he was three times my size. He whispered in my ear not to make a sound. I felt trapped, with no chance of escape.

My mind scrambled with confusion. What was happening to me? Then, in that moment of terror, I felt him put his penis inside of me. The pain was too much for me; I blacked out. I would later learn that what happened is clinically referred to as "splitting," which is a method children naturally use as a way of dealing with the pain associated with sexual abuse.

While my spirit was outside of my body, it was Our Heavenly Father who held me tenderly in His arms while my earthly body was being defiled by this less than human monster.

As I returned to my shivering, nude body, I felt my attacker's strong fingers—to me they were huge—tighten around my neck until I could hardly breathe. The terror and horror of what was happening to me returned instantly. His hot, sweaty mouth was next to my ear whispering, "If you tell anybody, I'll kill you, your mother, your sister, and your baby brother." With shallow breath and tears streaming down my cheeks, I heard my own tiny, weak voice say, "I won't tell. I promise." The terrifying secret would stay buried within me for over 30 years.

Like many sexually abused children, my attacker was a "friend" of the family, the teenage brother of my sister's girlfriend. Their house was the neighborhood place where all the kids wanted to hang out. The mother, for some reason, stayed hidden in her bedroom; the father spent long hours away at work. With no adult supervision, there were no rules to follow. We kids took over the house, eating junk food, jumping on furniture and staying up as late as we wanted.

After that terrifying night, I stopped wanting to go to their house, but Mom insisted that if my sister went, so did I. Fear of being molested again would grab my mind as I argued with my sister, trying to get out of going. Pressure from an older sibling is hard to fight, especially without being able to give the real reason; Max's threats of killing my family and molesting me scared me to death, so I always gave in. Sickeningly, Max molested me on a regular basis, no matter how hard I tried to hide amongst the other children on the living room floor at the hangout. I was terrorized, trapped and abused with no escape in sight.

Max was not the first to use my little body for his own pleasure. Two years earlier, my mother's boyfriend had taken me to his trailer and fondled me. Although he didn't threaten my family, my mother's overreaction to the situation sent me the wrong message. My mother was emotionally fragile, and even at the tender age of four I felt I had to protect her.

So when Max began to molest me, I silently endured his repeated attacks and prayed every night that my father would come back to save us. He was my hero, my knight in shining armor, my superman; he would end my horror. He never came. Unable to be a father, he had abandoned our family when I was two. It was his wild, selfish, drunken party lifestyle that took him away from us.

He did not pay child support, either. Back in 1959, not much was done to help women whose husbands abandoned them. Mom's family did little to help her, so, to feed her children, welfare was her only choice. As a result of mom trying to cope with it all, she slipped into depression. Even at that young age, I sensed what was happening to her; unable to tell anyone what was happening to me, feeling alone, and shouldering the added responsibility of protecting our family from Max's threats was overwhelming.

When I was a little older, a similar incident occurred within my own family. Jack was my cousin who had joined the Navy and was stationed in San Diego. He was the oldest cousin and my mother's favorite. Like her, he was born and raised in South Dakota, so Los Angeles was a completely different culture for him.

Many weekends when I was between the ages of 10 and 13, he would come and stay the weekend. He always slept on the couch in the living room. One morning I got up before the rest of the family. It was winter and the house was cold. He invited me to lie under the covers with him, which I naively did. He proceeded to put his hands all over my body. Flashing back to my experiences with Max, I froze and couldn't move, while he enjoyed himself all the way to ejaculation right there on the living room couch.

After that morning, when he came to visit I would stay in my room until the rest of the family was up, but he would walk by me and pretend to wrestle with me in front of the family, grabbing me in private areas. When I complained to my mother, she said that I was wrong and shouldn't say bad things about him.

Many years later, after my second divorce, he invited me to dinner. Having buried the fondling incidents, I went. Thank goodness I took my own car, because he lewdly suggested we become extremely close cousins. I got up and left the restaurant and have not seen him since that evening some 15 years ago. In 2004 my mother told me Jack was living in a homeless shelter, so there is some justice in the world!

Even though Mom was depressed, she was dating. At first, I thought her decision to marry Simon was a good one, a way out of my horror. I thought he was the answer to my prayers; he owned his own business and had five adult children, but what does an eight-year-old child know? My feelings soon changed; he sexually molested me one night shortly after their marriage and did what others had done before. The fear I had experienced with Max now turned into the same nightly horror as Simon waited for the rest of the family to fall asleep. He would then come into my bedroom and torture me with his sick demands.

Because as children we didn't have any spending money, when Christmas time came around Simon would offer to give us money if we sat on his lap and told him how wonderful he was as a father. Wanting to vomit, but wanting more to give our mother something special for Christmas, we would sit on his lap and tell him what he wanted to hear. To our surprise, right in front of our mother he would fondle us, and keep us there until he was done.

Almost worse than the sexual abuse were the mental and emotional torment Simon heaped upon me, my mother, and my siblings.

Simon had a twisted way of teaching us about life. One rare evening when I was about 12 years old, we were all at the kitchen table after dinner. I think something had happened at his job that pissed him off and he needed an audience to vent. Simon was talking about how we shouldn't trust other people outside the family. While he was expressing is deep seated opinions on this topic, he had a fork in hand, and said to me, "Jayne, put your hand on the table and spread your fingers." He kept talking about trust as he jammed the fork between my fingers. I was too scared to move; once again I was trapped. About this time he jammed the fork into my hand and

"If a child is unfortunate enough to be raised by an adult who is randomly abusive, the world becomes a frightening war zone for the child." Dr. Dave Ziegler and Michael Reaves compared young sexually abused children to war veterans. What they found was that "there are far more similarities than differences between veterans and [abused] children." The most notable and concerning difference is that children have an open wound. Because they are young and stuck in their environment — and therefore unable to control it — the abuser could strike at any moment, whereas veterans can rationalize an end to war, at which time they gain back control in their life. (Ziegler, 2000)

said, "Now that should be a lesson to you, don't trust anyone." Ever since then trust has been a major issue with me.

Simon came from the old school and believed that children were your property and you could do with them as you wished. When Mom married him, his gardening business was doing extremely well. He decided that during the summer he would have us kids go work for him on his route. My brother was too small and my older sister just flat out refused. So I was told I would be spending my summers working 12 hours days with him. That also included weekend special jobs, like mowing an entire vacant lot. However the grass was more like weeds and had to be pulled out by hand. Once that was done he would mow it, but the dirt was hard and the mowing created huge clouds of dust. I would have to follow him with a rake, piling up the dry hard grass. After 12 hours of that you go home dragging.

I complained about the hot sun, long hours, and the aches in my body. He told me that I was the "good" child and would be rewarded with money at the end of the summer. In many domestically violent environments, the children are pitted against each other so they don't form a united stand against the abuser. Survival is paramount. Your sibling has the power to bring the wrath of the monster down around your ears with a simple suggestion that you did something wrong.

I believed my father's promise and worked even harder each day, but the summer ended and the money never came. Not only did he fail to keep his promise, but he raided our small saving accounts to pay bills. When my sister and I complained, we were told how selfish we were and how HE was sacrificing to feed us. My summer lawn job continued until he closed his business and went to work at McDonnell Douglas.

For a few years while I was in junior high, Simon worked the graveyard shift. During the school year this was great because he would be gone to work when we got home from school, and would just be getting home as we were going to school. It never dawned on me until years later how horrible it was for my mother.

The exception was, of course, holidays, and summer vacation. During these days, while Simon slept in the house, Mom would take us kids to the garage and play all kinds of card games and board games with us. We all knew that anything would set him off, and either Matt, my younger brother, or Mom would get beaten for it, or the screaming and carrying on would be unbearable.

So to the garage we would go with the fold up table that he used on weekends when he would make us spend the day selling things at the swap meets while he pocketed all the money.

Never were we allowed to open up the large garage door for fear a neighbor would come over and start asking questions. So in the summer time it was sweltering hot and during the holiday vacations it was freezing cold.

Only now can I imagine the guilt my mother must have felt having her children as prisoners in the freezing/sweltering garage. The only thing distinguishing this from prison was the lack of bars. Or her horror when one of us would need to go into the house to use the restroom. Her terror each time we would open the door, fearing a squeak; the anxiety that gripped her body when we took longer to return than she thought was necessary, hoping that we didn't do anything that he would hear while we were in the house. Then her relief as we came back and took our places around the table, wrapping ourselves up in a blanket to keep warm.

This was followed, I am sure, by several minutes of sheer terror that at any second the monster who dwelled in our house would burst through the garage door to devour her or one of her children.

Once those terrorizing minutes had passed, the relief she must have felt when all was normal again. Normal for a 33 year old woman who sat with her children playing games in the sweltering heat or the freezing cold so they all would survive just one more day of terror.

As the years progressed, I was becoming more vocal in my opinions. Unbeknownst to me, Simon saw a determined, maturing child growing up. One way he thought he could control me was through mental and verbal abuse. He told me daily that I was stupid and ugly, and that no man would ever marry me.

Children only know what "normal" is from the adults around them. Normal for me was being sexually and mentally abused on a daily basis for the first 18 years of my life. These sexual acts are not normal for a child and my intuition told me they were wrong. To cope, many times I resorted to thought of Simon's death. In a crazy way, I felt this was the only way to handle the horror of those terrifying years.

Simon's control over the family made my sister and me beg our mother to leave. Her answer was always the same: She had made her bed, now she was going to stay and make the marriage work. Women of my mother's era did not have the choices we experience today.

When I finally reached 18, the plans my older sister and I envisioned for years of being together in our own apartment never materialized, as the man of her dreams came into her life. So I decided I wasn't going to move out of the house leaving my mother and brother to endure Simon's daily rage. However, my sister's wedding was the catalyst under which I found myself moving out. In fact, Mom was forbidden to go to the wedding. Simon didn't want me to attend the wedding either, but I did. When I returned home that night he demanded to know "everything that took place."

What came out of my mouth next shocked him and me equally; where I found the courage to say it is still beyond me. I stood up to him and said, loud and clear, "I won't tell you a damn thing. If you were a decent person, you would have been invited!" With fire in his eyes and a clenched fist, he took a step towards me, as he yelled, "I'll throw your ass through that plate glass door—you'd better start talking." I wouldn't realize the impact of what happened next for years to come. I took a step toward him and said, "It'd better kill me because if it doesn't, I'll have your ass thrown in jail!" I moved out the next day, leaving my little brother and mother behind.

It was two years later that the situation reached a

> "In 2000, home was not a safe haven for 2.7 million children across this great land of ours" (NCCAN). Abused children lived in terror every second of the day, wondering where the next blow, punch, kick or sexual advance would come from, be it father, mother, sibling, or so-called friend. 2,475 children are victims of this horrendous crime each day. "Tragically, an average of three children die every day as a result of child abuse or neglect. Each week, child protective services (CPS) agencies throughout the United States receive more than 50,000 reports of suspected child abuse or neglect" (NCCAN).

nightmarish height. Mother finally announced her intention to leave. It was then that Simon's rage reached a new pinnacle. Simon, being 6'2" to my mother's 5'2", was able to throw her down on the bed, point a gun in her face, and pull the trigger! If my brother hadn't previously taken the initiative to remove the bullets, my mother could have been killed. Mom and my brother did, in fact, leave with only the clothes on their backs. Everything else was burned by Simon in another fit of rage.

It was wonderful to finally escape my abusive environment, but terrifying at the same time. Terrifying because I realized I was "untaught," completely lacking in the life skills I needed to survive in this unfamiliar adult world in which I now found myself. Grateful, however, that through all the years of sexual abuse I did not become pregnant or contract a sexually transmitted disease, unlike so many other young girls whose lives are so much more complicated because of those outcomes. I had a job, but a checking account was beyond my understanding. I could eat, but it took time to learn to purchase healthy economical food. I didn't have an apartment, a car, savings or any understanding of what was happening to me. My interpersonal and social skills just didn't exist. It was because of the domestic violence environment in which we lived; outside people weren't allowed in for fear that the secrets would be found out. Like a felon released from prison, I was once again alone, lost, and scared in this "free" world in which I was now living.

Adulthood

Adulthood

Much to my sister's surprise, when she returned from her honeymoon, I was waiting on her front doorstep. She did let me sleep on their couch while I was trying to figure out what I was going to do with myself. As was understandable, my intrusion into their lives was less than a desirable situation for both her and her new husband.

As the weeks passed, they asked me daily what my plans were. I couldn't give them an answer. I was just trying to get through this situation, and without life skills to draw from, I was unable to formulate any kind of plans.

Sometime over the next two weeks, my new brother-in-law's cousin, Cliff, came by to "visit." What I didn't realize was that it was a date! Cliff had seen me at their wedding and wanted to get to know me. What we both didn't know on our first meeting is that he would become the "plan" that everyone was asking me about.

Marriage to Cliff was a way out of this difficult situation; my sister and brother-in-law didn't want me. I couldn't go back home. I had no money.

After 10 years of Simon telling me almost daily, "You are stupid, ugly, and no man would want to marry you!"

Cliff's marriage proposal was vindication that what Simon had said was not true.

When my first son was born 11 months later; I was 19; his brother arrived 18 months after that. The marriage was doomed from the start. It never occurred to me that Cliff might not be the man for me. We fought daily over his inability to keep a job, and his refusal to watch our boys while I worked. His mother supported his lack of responsibility by giving him money which he gambled away at the racetrack. By 21, I was divorced.

In between the births of my first two sons, I decided to find my biological father, Bill. From age two to age 19, I hadn't heard from my father, nor did I have a picture of him. I knew he had been a Navy Seal and had married many times, but had no idea where to start looking for him. I was living in Southern California; he ended up being closer than I thought, in Northern California just east of San Francisco.

Mom had given me the name of his sister, Sue. I found her phone number and, when I called, her ex-husband answered. As it turned out, Aunt Sue was having a "new procedure" — triple bypass surgery — in three days. To my delight, my father was coming to visit her before her surgery.

As I walked into my aunt's hospital room, I got the shock of my life! Aunt Sue and I could have been mother and daughter. When my father walked in the room, he did a double-take upon seeing me standing at the foot of her hospital bed. I wasn't sure if it was because of our resemblance, or if it was just me. Needless to say, it was a very emotional reunion. Six months later, he and his wife moved to Los Angeles to be closer to my sister and me.

After my divorce from Cliff with no pre-planning, I was once again thrown onto an unknown playing field. My father let the boys and me stay with him for two weeks. This took me 40 miles away from my job, so I quit, not realizing that with just a high school education and limited work experience—six months at K-Mart and a year in an office—and the two boys, ages three and one, I couldn't find a job. On top of all that, the fights with Cliff became uglier.

With my lack of parenting skills and the confusion going on in my life, my oldest son started to "react" to the situation. This caused a major problem with baby-sitters; I couldn't keep them. He would create total havoc in the day care and the sitter would greet me at the door at night to say, "Don't bring him back tomorrow." This happened three times in one week with three different baby-sitters. I kept losing jobs, so I decided to live on the $200.00 a month child support I was getting from Cliff. What else could I do? I lived in day-to-day crises without the skills to understand and solve my problems.

Now, most parents who are watching their adult daughter and two small grandsons going through our daily crises would do something to help: offer advice, baby-sit, give a little money, help with the bills or simply feed us. Bill's answer to the situation was, he would become my *PIMP!* He literally approached me one day and explained his connections in Hollywood with the taxi cab drivers. He would watch my boys while I was working the streets of Hollywood, California.

I had only known Bill for two years; I learned that he had fathered eight children, which resulted in his not being around to see any of us grow up or pay child support. We did know he ran an illegal gambling operation out of L.A. while owning a furniture store, and that he was an alcoholic, and still loved my mother.

No other help was offered after Bill made his disgusting suggestion. It must have been the look on my face of "I'd go to hell first."

I went out and found a paper route in the hills of L.A. This way I could take the boys with me in the car and deliver the paper to the mansions that comprised my route.

As my life was starting to move in the right direction, mom finally decided to leave Simon. She and my brother moved into our two-bedroom apartment with the boys and me. Mom, who was broke and hadn't worked in 10 years, got a job right away at a discount store. I thought everything was great and moving in a forward direction once again until the phone call!

I was living in the same apartment building as Bill and wife number six. Bill called Mom and asked her out on a date! Talk about role reversal. I refused to let him talk to her. So he came over anyway! About a month later, they moved in together with my brother.

Think my life got better? Well, think again. Turns out wife number six "knew" the owner of the apartment building before Bill married her. So she got the owner of the building to evict the boys and me.

What did my parents do for the us? Nothing! My boyfriend at the time had an uncle who owned a 100-year-old home. Just hours before I was to move, I literally begged my boyfriend's uncle to let the boys and me live there until I could get on my feet. That lasted 90 days; when I broke up with the boyfriend, his uncle asked me to move. However, being 40 miles away from my paper route, I quit that job and again became unemployed.

I was once again living on the $200-a-month child support and didn't have a clue what I was going to do next. It was suggested that if I could manage an apartment building, I could have a place to live. I figured I could do anything if given a chance. So I became the manager for a 10-unit apartment building in Van Nuys, California. This sounded good to me because I wouldn't have to leave the boys with anyone, and we could live on property. I took the job.

I gave the boys the only bedroom in our tiny, one-bedroom apartment and put a mattress in the dining room for myself. A three-legged kitchen table and a TV whose picture offered only shadows were the only furniture I owned. Rent, with the discount for managing, was $75.00. To earn extra money, I cleaned and painted filthy apartments.

However, as you can imagine, $200 a month for all the needs of a family of three wasn't making it, so when there were no apartments to clean, the boys and I would walk down Van Nuys Boulevard in the San Fernando Valley, digging in trash cans for food and collecting pop bottles to redeem for cash.

What a sight I must have been, standing by the entrance to the grocery store, counting and recounting the loose change in my hand with my two beautiful boys beside me. After carefully analyzing the food I had plucked from the trash, and satisfied that I had the proper amount of change to purchase the remainder of the food I needed for the week, I would lead my little family into the store. With an eagle eye on the cashier's entries, we'd stand at the checkout counter with our

17

shoulders back, our heads held high, and smiles on our faces. Looking back, everyone must have recognized our situation, but I was too proud to let anyone feel sorry for us. We lived this way for a year. Life was good, the fighting with the ex had settled down and I was with my sons all day.

It was the first time in my life that I can remember having a plan (if you can recall digging in trash cans a plan) and feeling like I was on a positive road. But it wouldn't last long.

At the age of 23, another unsuspecting man asked me to marry him. Dick was a member of the church I was attending. He was 13 years older than I and had a job. He also came with two children, Jennifer, 13, and Ron, 10. Dick's ex-wife sent the children to live with us three months after we married. At 24, I gave birth to my third precious son, and at 26, my fourth precious son was born. In my tender mid-twenties, I was the proud mother of four sons and two stepchildren.

Before I reached 30, I felt 80, and with that came the overwhelming feeling that my life was over. Despite the child abuse, the divorce, and even struggling to make a living for the two boys and myself, I had never been truly depressed until then. There was no end in sight. My life was not my own. Instead, it was dishes, laundry, dirty diapers, spilt milk, car-pooling, trips to the ER, participation in a male-dominated church, and other people often living with us. After years and years of this, Jayne was nowhere to be found. I had simply vanished.

I became incredibly anxious. Often I couldn't breathe because of these feelings of terror with nothing familiar or normal to fall back on. It wasn't the fear that I had come to know for 18 years, it was a different kind of fear that I was ill prepared to handle. Where was I going to sleep tonight? How was I going to get to work? I didn't know!

Dick's idea of a good marriage was: "I work outside the home for 40 hours a week, you do everything else." So when the wind and rain came and ripped shingles off our roof, I was up there fixing it the best way I knew how. It was divine intervention when the next night, I woke up and moved the children from their beds. A couple of hours later, the ceiling caved in on the very bed where they had been sleeping. Once again my Heavenly Father stepped in and saved us.

I stayed, trying to handle everything myself to avoid a second divorce. But the hole was getting deeper, and I was starting to sink. I thought maybe if I prayed more, read more scriptures, volunteered more at our church, I would find the answer. After all, that's what the church leaders and my husband were telling me. So I took on more responsibilities at the church by becoming the president of the 189-member women's organization—a position that added 20-plus hours of work to my already overwhelming schedule. Sheer survival instinct led me to develop a series of very effective organizational and time management skills.

Sundays, for me, consisted of 10 hours of meetings. While I was doing the Lord's work at church, Dick was at home napping and snacking. I'd most often return home to crying, starving children. When I confronted him, his comeback was, "Well, you should've gotten something ready for them before you left. You'd better pray more about your inability to organize yourself!" As he talked, the old recording played in my head: "You are stupid, ugly, and no man will marry you." The hole grew ever deeper, and I slipped further into it.

Just like during my childhood, deep down inside, I knew there was a major problem in my life. But I had no one to talk to. I had no idea how to handle all that I had experienced. As a child, being raised in a home of domestic violence, I was not allowed to have friends. So it stands to reason that as an adult, still under a domestic violence umbrella, I was conditioned not to talk to anyone about my problems. Because I was in charge of the 189-woman organization in our church, I was considered the number one woman in our church. Most of the church members assumed that our marriage was "perfect;" I thought I had no one to turn to.

Then one day, while folding mountains of clothes and towels in front of the TV, I saw a story about a 55-year-old nun who had begun long-distance running. To an over-worked, depressed woman like me, this woman looked ancient. But there she was, doing something she had waited to do for over 35 years. Not only was she running, she was winning. It was the ray of hope I needed to start gaining control of my life. I started my first "dream list" of things I wanted to do at each stage of the kids' lives. The very first thing on that list was to get my tubes tied. NO MORE CHILDREN!

It was also at this time in my life that I realized knowledge was the key to getting out of this hole that I was in. I read and read and read books on every subject you can imagine: history, mystery, science, courtroom dramas, etiquette, and art were just a few of the subjects I was drawn to. Biographies were and are still my favorite; the subjects, people past and present, became mentors in my mounds-of-dirty-diapers world. I was often reading five different books at any given time — I couldn't seem to absorb enough knowledge. I developed a love for books that would be the catalyst for my escape.

When I took the kids to Little League, pre-school, and doctors' offices, I took along my books. They fed the hungry beast inside of me. Soon, I started taking the kids to museums, concerts, and fine restaurants to teach them what I was learning. I felt, for the first time in my life, as if I were heading down a path where I could see the light at the end of the tunnel. In addition, I had gotten a job, which gave us a newfound level of comfort. Unfortunately life, as it will, was about to toss me a major curveball.

The black hole sucked me in deeper after visiting my terminally ill father-in-law in the hospital. While I was driving my mother-in-law home, she announced she couldn't take the stress any longer. She was filing for divorce; he would be our responsibility now. My mother-in-law's utter lack of Christianity shook me to my very soul. At this time, besides the boys we had another family of four living with us, but we took my father-in-law into our home with open arms. We set him up in the front bedroom; we then condensed the rest of the family into two back rooms. Naturally, I assumed that Dick would help care for his dying father, but he wouldn't even acknowledge that his own father was in our home.

Regardless, I wouldn't give up. Every day, I was up at 4:00 a.m. saying my prayers, reading my scriptures, taking care of my father-in-law, getting the school lunches made, reviewing homework, organizing the house, starting laundry, preparing for the women's organization, taking out the trash, getting the boys up for school, and heading off to work by 5:00 a.m.

In fact, work ended up serving as my five-day-a-week escape from home. By 2:00 p.m., I would head for home, arriving about 3:00, and once I hit the door it all started again. There were doctor appointments, shopping, dinner by 4:00, yard work, homework, Little League practice, conferences with teachers, canning, dehydrating, sewing; the to-do list never ended. I collapsed in bed every night from sheer exhaustion, only to be awakened a few short hours later by one emergency or another. Dad would need to be rushed to the hospital, or I would simply need to calm his fears about dying alone. While holding his hand, I listened to the stories of his life, his regrets, and his sorrows. The only thing that would slow me down was a van that broke on such a regular basis that the tow-truck drivers knew me by name. At Christmastime, I gave them homemade cookies and candy. Even though I was doing all these things, I still felt like the hole was swallowing me.

Another ray of hope came when the vice president of the company I was working for saw my potential and suggested I go into sales. The very thought was overwhelming. Up until then I had only worked to make money, not to have a career. Before I realized what was happening, I had found a mentor in my boss. She would give me the tools I needed to change my life dramatically.

In sales I thrived. I was paid what I was worth, I learned how to set real goals and accomplish them, and most importantly, my self-esteem started to grow; this domino effect created other changes in my life. I was now out in the gentile world, seeing and talking to people other than just the church members. I started to question the church, my marriage, and, more than ever before, my life.

This period marked the beginning of the end of my second marriage. I began to realize that although he didn't kick or punch, Dick's control over me was domestic violence. Still, that old recording played in my head, "...stupid, ugly, no man will marry you..."

During the time my father-in-law lived with us he asked me never to put him in a rest home. The doctor took it out of my hands on November 5th when he would not release my father-in-law to my care, but sent him to a convalescent home.

Feeling that I sentenced my father-in-law to death was the final straw that sent me to the mountaintop! While driving on this winding canyon road, I thought to myself, "If this is what life is about, I don't want to live anymore!" Instead of making the next turn, I pushed the accelerator to the floor and pointed the car straight for the edge of the mountain. Incredibly, some unknown force applied the brakes and the car stopped, just inches from the edge. I sat and cried uncontrollably.

Realizing I had almost committed suicide, I called my bishop; he suggested I call our church counselor. The counselor explained that there wasn't any way to fit me into his schedule for the next two weeks. It must have been the way I said "okay," because his next question was, "Jayne, describe to me how you are feeling right now."

"Well," I said, "I am on the inside of a black, bottomless hole. I am holding onto the edge and my fingers are starting to slip." I was in his office within the hour.

In counseling, it was determined that my husband wasn't supporting me emotionally. The counselor described me as being a water well, but my well was so dry from lack of support from anyone that there were major cracks in the bottom of it.

For two years, while going through therapy, Dick wouldn't acknowledge that there was a problem with our marriage, nor did he support me, despite what the counselor had said. Instead, he told me over and over again that I was going to hell for not praying hard enough. He arranged for me to be hauled off to be judged by higher authorities in the church where I was told that I was "satanic" for not following the word of my husband. I wondered why my loving Heavenly Father would want me to be miserable. Was He pushing me to the point that I didn't want to live? I think not. I filed for two divorces: one from my husband and one from the church.

While going through the divorce from Dick, I decided to move with the boys back to Orange County, California, where I was raised. It was closer to my family and to the beach. My hope was to get help with the boys, rent out our family home in the Valley and maybe get an education for myself. The sales position at the Cally Curtis Company was going extremely well; the only downside would be my morning commute into Hollywood which would increase from 20 miles to 50 miles one way, I felt it was worth the extra time on the freeway to be close to family.

Dick and I had purchased the house in 1976 for $47,500, and a real estate agent said I could get $248,000 for it. Even with the first and second mortgages totaling $87,500 I was happy -- until the contractors started giving me their open ended bids.

In order to rent the house I would have to hire contractors to fix everything Dick hadn't done over the last 13 years. After 5 contractors inspected it, it was determined that the house was a disaster. Termites had eaten out the main beam, the roof leaked in several places, and the two additions flooded every year. There was dry rot and mildew all around the bottom of the walls.

Contractors came and went, all refusing to give me a closed bid; they wanted to rip out drywall to see what the real damage was. The bids started at $75,000 and went up from there. I was overwhelmed, pissed, and devastated.

In addition to the contractors, my attorney fees were going through the roof. After agreeing to everything in court, Dick wouldn't sign the divorce papers. He fired his attorney and hired another one. This was interesting since his first attorney did all the work at no cost. Anyway, this forced me back into court. The reason he took me back to court was that I'd gotten the house in the divorce. He didn't want more time with the kids, he didn't want lower child support, he didn't want to keep me in the same county. He wanted the house.

In addition to the contractors, and Dick pulling me back into court, the church I had attended for 17 years decided I was satanic, and shouldn't have my children. Several women in the church worked in the schools my sons attended. I started getting calls from the school psychologist; he wanted to meet with me to discuss the emotional stability of my children. The meeting consisted of the school principal, psychologist, and the teacher of my youngest son, then 9 years old. They asked me a series of questions like: Are you going through a divorce? Is there a man other than the sons' father living there? When do you go to work? When do you get home? Do you spank your children?

After they asked all their questions I asked a few of my own. Are the boys' grades slipping? Are they disrupting the class? Who is bringing my children to your attention?

To my surprise, they named the women who said the school should check into my family. It was the women in the church. The very women to whose homes my sons would go to play. The very women to whom I took food when they were sick. The very women I stood next to at the church socials dishing out food.

I felt betrayed, I felt bewildered, I felt furious!

I demanded to know what exactly this panel of "educators" was looking for. Here is what caused them to pull me in and "talk" with me. On school picture day my youngest son wore a ripped shirt, his hair was not combed, and his jeans were dirty. As they were reading this short list, I braced myself for the big stuff to come. Instead they stopped talking. I waited a minute then said, "anything else?"

"No" was the response.

My anger grew, but somehow I managed to keep my cool. Looking each person right in the eye I said, "My son is 9 years old. I am at work at 6 a.m. so his older brothers, ages 11 and 14, help get him dressed. The shirt he wore on picture day is his favorite, and I didn't sew it. Now you tell me how many boys this age are going to comb their hair by themselves? My neighbor also has a son his age and she watches the boys each morning to make sure they get off to school on time. Furthermore, the reason I go to work at 6 a.m. is so I can be home by 3 p.m. to be with my sons, who as you know get out of school at 2:30 p.m. Unless you have something else you haven't talked to me about I am leaving. The next time you pull me in to talk about my sons be ready to meet my attorney. This is harassment."

While all this was going on my friend Laura decided I needed a break; she wanted me to go to Palm Springs for a weekend. When we were all ready to go she announced that her brother-in-law was the assistant general manager at one of the hotels there. I told her I didn't want to get involved with another man right then. She promised me that wasn't the reason we were going.

However, to people living in L.A., Palm Springs was the place married people went to have affairs. All I needed was for my soon to be ex-husband to find out I went to Palm Springs and stayed at my friend's brother - in- law's hotel. I didn't go.

My friend then invited me to Thanksgiving Dinner, and I accepted. The boys would be with their fathers, and I would be alone. A couple of days later I found out that her brother-in-law would be there. I didn't show up or even call to say that I wouldn't be coming.

Now very unhappy with me, she asked me to come to Christmas dinner, and because I felt guilty I both accepted her invitation and showed up. Albert, her brother-in-law, had just come out of alcohol rehabilitation. At first we both were stressed out, because of our current situations.

After that Laura would arrange for the two of us to meet at her house. He moved from Palm Springs to Marina de Ray, which was only 10 miles from Hollywood, where I worked. I started leaning on him for support as I was going through all the stress. One day I stopped by his office on my way home, to talk to him about Laura's upcoming surprise birthday party.

All of a sudden I got dizzy to the point where I had to lie down. Things didn't get better so he took me to his apartment. Laura stayed with the kids. The next day I was at the doctor's office, but he had no idea what was going on. The dizziness was getting worse, not better, as each day passed. I was freaking out because I hadn't been home in two days. After a week I went to a neurosurgeon to try and figure out what was going on. They never did find out what was wrong, but decided it was all the stress I was under and gave me antidepressants. At first I refused to take them, but the doctor explained to me that I was on a dangerous road and needed some relief. Up until that point in my life, even with all that I had been through I never drank or used drugs. I was not happy, but needed to be able to function.

While all of these things were going on in my life, Albert was there. After the boys went to bed, he would call me and just listen. One day he asked if he could take the boys and me camping. The boys loved it and I felt I needed to get away more often as the divorce and the house were moving slowly forward.

During these camp-outs I told Albert all of the dreams and goals I was setting down for myself. We talked well into the night as the boys were sleeping. He was easy to talk to and agreed with all that I said. After several weekends like this he popped the question: Did I want to go to Palm Springs with him for the weekend? I never was a person to sleep around, so this question was a very serious question to me. After days of thinking about his offer, I accepted.

Deep down, I think I was tired of handling all these issues all at once and by myself, so I gave up and gave in. Five months after my divorce was final Albert and I were married in Las Vegas. Six months after that we moved to Orlando, Florida.

From the day we stepped foot into Florida, he reverted to the individual he really was -- someone I did not recognize. I was shocked and angry. We had talked for hours. I had painstakingly explained to him what I wanted in life and he had wholeheartedly agreed. He said he could live with it; he lied. I wanted to go to a marriage counselor. He refused.

For the first 9 months he didn't work. One day he would say I was wonderful the next that I was stupid. In California he couldn't get enough of the boys, but in Florida he barely spoke to them. Another huge issue came up and that was our sexual relationship. Once in Florida he didn't want to have sex any longer. I was told I

What the counselor had missed, and what I didn't yet understand, were the patterns of behavior I had developed in childhood that I was still following. Although headed in a positive direction, without realizing it, I was still listening to the same voices in my head, particularly when it came to choosing a spouse. When Albert asked me to marry him, the same old recording was still playing in my head. "You are ugly, stupid and no man would want to marry you." In marrying Albert and moving to Florida, I was hoping a new husband and new surroundings would fix everything that had gone wrong in my adult life. I still didn't understand that I was the one with the problem.

caused him to be impotent. During the day he would say that night would be the night, then that night he would say, no. Living with him was a roller coaster ride, and my self esteem plummeted.

A recovering alcoholic with whom I worked explained to me that Albert's behavior suggested that he was a dry drunk, a recovering alcoholic who doesn't drink. But the roller coaster ride was the same as if he were drinking.

Once again realizing I had made a big mistake, I was devastated, but this time I was trapped in Florida. I had accepted a sales position to work from home as an independent contractor, selling training videos for The Telephone Doctor. Both situations -- working from home and being self-employed -- being totally new to me, I was ill-prepared to handle them plus this new husband who had turned out to be someone else I didn't know.

Feeling trapped again, I started trying to figure out what to do now that I was 3,000 miles away from friends and family, and faced with a job market that didn't pay what I was accustomed to earning. Time passed quickly, and before I knew it, two years had gone by.

I was preparing to divorce Albert when life took me on yet another journey that would change my life forever. On Friday, Oct. 2, 1992, while driving home from a business meeting during a monsoon rain on the Courtney Campbell Causeway between St. Petersburg and Tampa, Florida, a driver lost control of her car and hit me. My car spun around and another car hit me head-on at 60 miles per hour. Para-medics took the woman who caused the accident, the man who hit me head-on, and me to the hospital, and tow-trucks took our cars to the auto graveyard. The causeway was closed, helicopters circled overhead, and we were on the 6 o'clock news.

Black and blue from head to foot, with a bruised kidney and a back that remains 25% damaged to this day, were the final straws that broke me, and opened up many years of secrets. I was emotionally, mentally and physically drained. I wanted to run away. A month later, I did run away and didn't return until I had a promise from Albert that we would see a marriage counselor.

A day later, in the counselor's office, I told my side of the story with all the vigor of a wildcat. Ann, the counselor, nodded her head and took notes. When it was Albert's turn, he got a funny look on his face, and then turned to me and said, "Jayne, I am sorry." Turning back to the counselor, he uttered the terrifying sentence I had been avoiding for over 30 years. "I think what Jayne is experiencing right now is somehow a result of being sexually molested as a child."

Instantly, I felt I couldn't breathe. I rose from my chair and the room started spinning. My brain was scrambled, my mouth was open, but I could not speak. My entire body shook. Before I could calm myself down enough to attack him, Ann looked at me and asked, "Is there any validity to what Albert just said?"

I turned my attention to her, and with fire in my eyes, but a stern, steady voice, I said, "Yes, but I will not talk to you about it. Do I make myself clear?" Then, in an instant, I was a frightened little girl. Turning to Albert, I said, "Now you've done it. Max is going to kill my family because you told. He told me not to tell. You just killed my family!" Raising my knees to my chest, I sat there for several minutes, shaking and sobbing uncontrollably.

The decision was made that I would see Ann three days a week to help me overcome my terrifying childhood history. In short order, I realized that I would have to relive what had happened, emotionally, physically and mentally, so I could purge it from the place inside my heart where it had been buried all those years.

Two weeks later, on a cold November day, while Albert was at work and the boys were in school, I calmly and methodically planned my own death. My irrational thinking was that I had lived through the pain and torment of the abuse once, why did I have to go through it again? Why did my children have to suffer because of what those inhuman bastards had done to me? I thought my sons would have a better chance of a normal life without me.

By the grace of God, I shared my suicide plan with my therapist. I thought my plan was a solid one, but she found holes in it. I went home and reorganized, but Ann just found more holes. We played this dangerous game for a couple of weeks. Then, one day I walked into Ann's office with bold confidence and announced, "I have made a decision." She held her breath. "Those bastards took my childhood, but I will not let them take any more of my adulthood. I hope you are good at what you do, because you hold the most precious thing in my life... ME! My family and I are depending on you and your skills. Let's fix me!"

When I made the commitment to Ann not to remove myself from the face of the earth, I feared that somehow I would not be "Jayne" once Ann got done with me. What she suggested was that Jayne was lost and together we would find her.

The journey would be long, difficult, and even terrifying at times; however the end result was something I had secretly dreamed of for 39 years. All those years, I knew I was different. I felt now I was unique, I was Jayne!

The very first thing Ann did was take away my dependence on list-making so I could get in touch with my feelings. It hurts so bad to be a victim, all I wanted to do is stop the pain, both physical and mental. In order to heal from these horrid memories I must go though the pain again to get to the other side. Realizing that I barely made it through the first time, an overwhelming fear set in that told me there is no way I could relive those experiences.

I was a child who couldn't protect herself; and I wondered whether I had the strength to protect myself now. Too overwhelmed to make this decision I said this prayer: "Heavenly Father, I can't do this anymore. I don't know what to do, please take this from me." And he did.

He sent me to Ann, who gave me the keys to live life to its fullest. However, this can not be done until you heal from the past. Karol Truman wrote a great book called, *Feeling Buried Alive Never Die.* I don't care what Aunt Bertha says about "don't bring up the past it only hurts others." Or "grow up and get over it." Or "he really didn't mean anything by it." The hell he didn't! I am here to tell you your Aunt Bertha was wrong, because I buried my childhood trauma so deep that it took three bad marriages, a trip to a mountain top, and a major car accident to bring me down.

With every fiber of my being I can tell you that you will not gain control of your life, create your dreams or live life to its fullest until you heal from the past. This doesn't mean, however, that you spend the rest of your life pointing fingers and feeling sorry for yourself.

It means that these issues are soooooo difficult to deal with that a professional psychologist, who is trained to help you, needs to be by your side. For years after I went through therapy I won't even tell people the name of the book and workbook I used, because if I hadn't had Ann to guide me through them, I personally believe I would have carried out my plan to end my life.

Many of you who have been abused sit in your house wrapped in fear, while the bad guys win again because now they have taken your adulthood. It's up to you to stop the cycle.

Most health care plans offer several visits to a psychologist or therapist to help you decide what is best for you. With professional help and support from friends and family you will be able to stand tall and take back which is yours. Your life.

In this healing process, anger would be the first emotion to explode. According to the workbook which Ann had given me, the most logical and appropriate response to abuse is anger. So it was normal for this to be the first "feeling" emotion for me to work through. Passive all my life, I was ready to do actual physical violence to my tormentors, and I knew how to use a gun.

Ann set down some ground rules I had to follow through this stage. I was not allowed to kill anyone. To my dismay, I really did want to kill these monsters, and plotted each of their deaths in graphic detail. Not being able to follow through with these plans created yet another stress in my life.

One day as I was trimming the bushes in the backyard, I strong-armed one limb, pulled it out as far as it would come, yelled Max's name at the top of my lungs, and "cut off his penis!" Within 10 minutes, the entire three-foot-tall, two-foot-wide bush was lying at my feet, and I felt victorious. The next day when I told Ann, she laughed and suggested that was a great way to deal with my bottled-up anger. From then on, as we began each session her first question would be, "How many bushes have you mutilated since we've seen each other?" Twenty-four bushes later, I got past the anger stage.

Realizing what had happened to me during my childhood and who had caused it was just the beginning. Broken down, beaten up, and exhausted, I was now going to move into fixing me, which is not an easy task for a 39-year-old mother of three teenage boys with a bad marriage and no job. It was impossible for me to work during the six months of intense therapy. Staying alive was my first and foremost goal in the early stage; many of those days I wouldn't come out of the bedroom, much less go look for a job.

Over the course of the next several months, Ann taught me the keys to handling the nightmares, depression, abandonment, anger, emotions, fear and anxiety. She taught me about feelings, being true to myself, and learning to say "no." She helped me understand why my parents couldn't and didn't protect me. She gave me permission to forgive or not forgive. While in counseling I learned how to trust my instincts, love myself even when I fail, and go after what I want in life, not what others want to hand me.

I remember when my youngest son signed up for baseball in the spring of 1993. He asked me if I would go watch him play. I had been in therapy for four months by then and decided it was time to "come out." The fear and anxiety I went through to just go to the baseball diamond was overwhelming to me. My fear of people took hold. It was all I could do to reply when another parent spoke to me. I didn't run away even though I wanted to... I was damned determined not to let those men, who took my childhood from me, take any more of my adulthood.

Albert loved me in his own way, but he had lied to get me to marry him. Once in Florida I think he thought I wouldn't leave because I had said I did not want another divorce. He kept me off center by his roller coaster rides. Now the boys were moving into their teenage years and creating many other challenges.

In therapy, I leaned to be honest with myself, to love me for me, and not try to control others. For the first time in my entire life I decided to take a break from divorce and marriage and all that comes with it.

This time I moved into another bedroom, and concentrated on healing me. That was fine with Albert, as he didn't want to have sex anyway. So for the next nine years we lived this way. The relationship turned from husband and wife to friends. We were both comfortable with this arrangement, until I gained self-confidence, lost weight, and started my own business.

He gained more weight, purchased guns, and went into a depression as he watched me soar. By this time I was in a Toastmasters club, and Albert in some crazy twisted way thought I was having affairs with all the men in the club. His jealousy became obsessive and frightened me. He demand I get my concealed weapons permit under the guise that when I traveled I would be protected. I had shot guns before and didn't have a problem with them, but the idea of shooting someone turned my stomach. Nevertheless, to keep the peace, I went with him to the classes.

On the first of the two-day class the instructor asked each one of us why we were getting a concealed weapons permit. When it was my turn, I said honestly, "My husband wants me to have it," which didn't set too well with the instructor. As the class progressed he could see that the thought of possibly killing someone was making me physically sick. Each time I would voice this, Albert would belittle and berate me. Finally the instructor couldn't take this any longer and stepped in to confront Albert. He told Albert to leave me alone, that this was my decision, not his. As I watched Albert, I could see the look of death in his eyes, and it shocked me into reality.

Albert's jealousy was getting worse as I was evolving into the woman who had been hidden inside me. We had gotten fat together, we had been together for over ten years, the boys were grown and gone, and I guess he figured I was over being mad about all of his lies. Our life together had gotten to the convenient stage. Even though we were not having sex, neither one of us looked out side the marriage for someone else.

The problem came in when I lost 75 pounds while he gained weight. I was developing my speaking talents and my day job was going extremely well; he lost his job. I am an extrovert, he was an introvert.

After the incident in the concealed weapons class, I started to review in my head all the comments, Albert had been making, such as "you are sleeping with all the men in your Toastmasters Club, you spend too much time at work" and "you want to spend more time with your sons than with me."

While all this was going on I decided to volunteer to speak at local businesses on behalf of Harbor House, Orlando's domestic violence shelter. In order to do this I went through a 3 hour orientation, which explained the patterns and personality types of abusers. Can you imagine my shock and surprise when, after reviewing the patterns and personalities, I saw Albert? I'm not saying he would have physically abused me but the path the two of us were headed down didn't promise a good ending for me. Another concern I had was that if he felt I was having an affair, instead of killing me, he might go after one of the guys in my Toastmasters Club or the businessman I worked with.

Armed with this realization, I knew I had to leave but was concerned that he might think I was leaving for someone else. So it took me six months of planting seeds with the idea we should go our separate ways. Finally he came to me and said, "I am not happy in this relationship; I think we should divorce." That was in about June of 1999; we stayed together for six more months to get everything worked out. In January of 2000 I moved into the cutest apartment over a garage in downtown Orlando. I was free!

When I went into heavy therapy to rid myself of all the demons, what a shock it was for me to realize that the biggest demon of all was my mother. I hated her for what she had allowed to happen to us. For allowing that monster to drive us to the garage, for beating my baby brother, for sexually molesting me, and in afflicting such mind control on my sister that it still affects her life today.

At first, in my mind she was the worst mother of all. She knew, she saw, she closed her eyes. Over two years passed as I tried to make some sense of it all. Why had she allowed her children to be abused? Why hadn't she gotten a job and moved out? We begged her weekly to do that. Did she love us? I mean *really* love us? If so how would she let that happen? These and so many more questions raced in my head for years.

After months of therapy and a lot of healing and growing had taken place, one day Ann, my therapist, said, "I want you to take a look at what your mother's life was like as a child, as a young woman, and as the mother you know her to be. I am not suggesting that she was right in her choices but I want you to look at her life the way we have been looking at your life these last few months."

At first the very idea that I would ever forgive her made me sick. How could I forgive what she had done to me!!! As I was thinking about what Ann had suggested I picked up the phone and called a few family members. I wrote down all that I knew about my mother's life as a child, as a young woman, and as my mother. I wrote letters to distant relatives asking general questions. I researched the eras in which she was a teenager, a young woman, young adult and middle aged woman. And here is what I uncovered after two years.

- She was the 5th child out of 6.
- She was the 4th girl out of 5.
- Her father was her idol.
- Her father was an alcoholic.
- He always had a job providing for his family.

- He was never at home, either working or in a bar.
- When he was at home she stuck by his side for protection.
- He told her secrets about himself that no one knew until the day he died.
- Her mother didn't like her and said so daily.
- She was accused of being dad's favorite.
- She was painfully shy and backwards.
- She couldn't spend a night away from home because she would get sick.
- Her sisters used this shyness to their advantage.
- She would escape into a book when her sisters teased her.
- She would be the only child in the family to finish high school.
- Her older sister died when she was younger.
- She was born in a town of 200 people in South Dakota.
- She was raised in a town of 500 people in South Dakota.
- She never had clothes that fit her properly because. the sister older than she was heavy and she was thin.
- Back then, being thin meant you were sick, so each day the teacher would make this shy little girl stand before the class and force cod liver oil down her throat until she gagged.
- She moved to the state capitol and got a job as a waitress.
- As a shy waitress she met Bill the cook.
- Bill and Mom married just a month later.
- Bill was already in a common law marriage. His wife's father was a politician and had Bill put in jail

for bigamy just as he and Mom came out of the Justice of the Peace after their wedding.

- She was embarrassed to go home but did so to explain the situation. She was ridiculed by everyone but her father, who helped get Bill out of jail.
- The jail deal meant Bill had to move to Chicago and he took his new bride hundreds of miles from home with no family.
- She hated Chicago.
- She had her first child in Chicago a long away from family and friends.
- Bill came home one day and told her he had joined the Navy and was moving to California.
- Bill had been raised in the L.A. area.
- She went home to South Dakota during his boot camp.
- Her first child developed allergies and almost died.
- Her mother fought with her about raising this sick child.
- Bill finally sent for her.
- She traveled by train by herself with 18-month-old daughter to Los Angeles Union Station.
- She hated California.
- For her, military life was rough.
- But she idealized Bill; he could do no wrong.
- Domestic violence starts in subtle ways: mostly mental.
- Bill partied and gave away their money.
- I was born during this time.
- Now there were two girls to raise.
- Bill was a Seal; he was always gone and she was alone.
- Her father died when I was 2, shocking her world.

- Bill openly had extramarital affairs, telling her she was no good.
- They divorced when I was 2 years old.
- She had no education.
- She tried to work but couldn't; I'm not sure why.
- Bill didn't provide child support.
- His family hassled her.
- She moved from family to family members' homes with two children dozens of times.
- They were of the opinion "you made your bed, now lie in it."
- The final blow came when I was 6 and she became pregnant out of wedlock in 1959.
- She went on welfare.
- When my younger brother was 2 she met Simon and got married.

Reading through this list, it was easier for me to understand that she really had no other choice but to marry Simon or at least, she didn't have anyone to help her or guide her. There were no support groups, there were no government run organizations to provide assistance, there were no welfare to work education programs, and her family got tired of her need of support. She did the best she could do with all that she had going on in her life. Was it a selfish move on her part? Was she lazy? Did she NOT love her children?

From the day they married she lived with a death threat, and she watched her children be abused mentally, physically, and sexually. There is no doubt in my mind that she was also being abused, because she would turn his anger to herself so that her children wouldn't get that round of abuse. She endured in silence for fear of death to her children. She died a little each day, witnessing what she did.

She was trapped with no end in sight. But she never gave up hope of getting her children out of the situation. She taught her children the value of an education, the value of following the ten commandments, the value of a good day's work. She sacrificed all that she ever wanted in life as an adult so food would be put on the table, so her children would be clothed each day, so they would not feel the rain and cold on their bodies.

When surviving there are no rules to follow. No one gives you a blueprint. In that day and time no one gave you a hand up. In fact, she was labeled as a scarlet woman when, in 1959, she became pregnant out of wedlock. I remember how proud I was that a little baby brother or sister was coming into our family. I was 6 years old and didn't realize how she must have died a thousand times standing in front of these adults who stood in judgment of her for being pregnant and single. But she never told me not to be proud of my brother.

When the welfare people came to deliver Thanksgiving dinner to us, how she must have cried that night, realizing she wasn't providing for her family and that she had no one to turn to. No one's shoulder to cry on. No one to hold her close and make it all right for even a few minutes. So when Simon came into her life she could see no other way.

Through a lifetime of faith, communication, and belief in my Heavenly Father, I eventually came to terms with those predatory men who had caused me so much pain, and with the mother who failed to protect me from them. After years of tormented prayers, I was trying to understand why they had done what they had to an innocent child. This question came to me: "How will those men justify to God what they did come Judgment Day?" Ann is the angel whom the Heavenly Father sent to me to save my life. For that I will be eternally grateful to both Him and her.

What follows in the rest of this book is a guide for you to follow to empower yourself. We're all different, so what worked for me may not work for you. Instead, of cutting bushes to get over the anger, you may break windows or write poems to express those emotions. The point is, A Wallflower No More is a guide to get you pointed in the right direction. The road you take will be up to you.

Ready to move on? Using one of my wonderful husband's sayings, "Let's get it done!"

Ripping at my Heart

*Rip, zip, pull, push… Tearing at the innermost core of my
    soul.*
There you are, there you go.
*All the while in my heart, in my mind, in my being,
    washing through my blood like a waterfall – flowing
    fast, strong, violent, soothing.*
All at once,
I drop – to my knees.
*Exhausted, out of breath, disoriented, feelings rushing, no
    feeling at all.*
Terror, shame, panic, disgust.
Where did it all go?
*Like a tornado that came in and ripped my life from under
    me.*
My foundations – gone.
Dust is all that remains.
*Shambled, wrecked, I try to stand – only to fall back to my
    knees.*
I cry out.
*Only a groan leaves my lips, for I know not of what I am
    even crying out for anymore.*
Hope almost gone in the midst of the disaster.
*I cling on to something – faith out there in the thick dust
    from which I used to see light through.*
Now there is only darkness, dark dust darkness.

Faith? Are you still there? Do you exist? Did you ever?
Another groan…
And, I fall hard – on my face.
Deep, deep I fall into a sleep after much hysteria, exhausted
from the tears, pain in my throat from the dry
coughing.
Much time passes and the morning sun rays awake me…a
faint voice I hear in the distance…
Is it in my mind? No…It's getting louder now…
My Father…my Father in Heaven has heard my cries.
He's telling me now to rest in His care.
"Will there be more pain?" I ask?
"Yes." He replies.
"Will you be there with me?"
"Yes," He confirms.
"Will it be scary?"
"Yes," He repeats.
And, then I hear, "With all your heart, trust in me and not
in your own judgment. The plans I have for you are
good."
I take a deep breath and lift my body. The weight which felt
almost unbearable last night feels a little lighter now.
"Okay," I say. "I will trust in you…for you are all I have
left now."

By Michelle L. La Vigueur

Employment

Employment

Because I moved so much and had so many children, I never stayed with a company very long.

The result was that I had low self esteem regarding work. The way I tried to compensate for it was through working extra hard, putting in longer hours with no pay, and doing personal things for my bosses.

A good example is the first job I got after 5 years of staying home with the children. It was a receptionist/front office position. The company tested circuit boards. I didn't realize how well I was doing this job until one day about 6 months into it I realized the office manager played all day and I did her work. I was organized, accurate with the bookkeeping, and kept all the balls up in the air during the day. And when the boss yelled at me to get his coffee which was in his office, I did it without question. After all I was nobody; I had been at home for 5 years.

A position came open as the customer service assistant. I went to the boss asking to be considered for the position. He said "yes, it's yours." The next day he promoted someone else. When I asked why he said the office manager had told him I was doing a great job where I was and she didn't want to lose me.

Within a month I quit, taking the customer service assistant position at the Cally Curtis Company, which produced training videos. After two weeks the vice president asked me to go into sales. I said no, than reconsidered after a month, and took the position. I felt so under qualified I was nervous that he had made a mistake letting me try this. I didn't dawn on me that he saw something in me that I had no idea was there. The new sales manager had eight years experience selling training videos, and took me under her wing. I listened and did everything she told me to do. The first thing was to watch each of our 40 training videos, and be able to tell a customer about them.

I diligently watched and re-watched each title on subjects like time management, customer service, organization skills, sales, how to manage people, how to handle multiple bosses, etc.; the subjects seemed to be endless. Within a month or two I could repeat word for word what was said in each video, and tell a customer what each scene was about. It took me about six months to become the top sales person, which is were I stayed the rest of my five years with the company, becoming the sales manager when my boss left.

Although I had accomplished this feat, being the top sales person in a short period of time, my self-esteem was still low, (not to mention that I was going through the second divorce with all its challenges) and I didn't feel I was doing a good enough job. I decided to take my training a few steps further. Then I learned about personality types, how to talk on the phone (we were inside sales people), how to close a sale, how to organize my time, how to make 300 phone calls a day. I read books on how to market our videos and on how to ask the customer what he wanted in training videos. I went to two trade shows a year with the company, so I learned how to sell at a trade show, and how to meet customers face to face.

All this training took place over the five years I worked for the company. When I announced in 1990 that I was leaving the Cally Curtis Company and moving to Florida, I had nine job offers from other training companies to work for them. Those nine job offers were my first clue of my capabilities. For the first time in my life, people around me were validating that I was smart, teachable, and able to do what I set my mind to.

Seven years later, I was working for Adverting On Hold (AOH), a small company that sold on-hold messages to organizations such as Darden Restaurants, Marriott Hotel, and the apartment industry nationally. During my time at AOH, I decided I wanted to start my own company with a friend. We started TJ Seminars in 1997, and the plan was for me to leave AOH in 1999. In addition, Albert and I decided to divorce, so between my own business, and selling advertising for Advertising On Hold, I was busy but happy.

In 1999, Advertising On Hold was purchased by another company. The owner had started AOH out of his garage 10 years earlier, and it had grown so successfully that now Muzak, the company that provides background music for offices, restaurants, hotels, etc. all over the country, wanted to purchase us. Now I was free to run my own business full time.

The boys were now on their own, but the bad news was that two lived in Southern California and two lived in Central Florida. So, my idea was to have my professional speaking business in Florida, and do speaking engagements in both California and Florida. The apartment industry was really a hot market for me at that time with respect to selling for Advertising on Hold.

As I was putting this together, Muzak came in and purchased AOH, as previously mentioned. And to my surprise they asked me to become the Sales Manager for the 5 current sales people, plus the additional 7 sales people they were hiring. I was shocked, to say the least, when they more than doubled my income.

It was a very hard decision because of my own personal business plans. After many trips to the beach and a long conversation with my partner, I decided to take TJ Seminars a bit slower, but keep her alive, and accept the sales manager position.

Between cutthroat managers, power hungry men and women, and lies that shocked me daily, the year I spent with Muzak could, in fact, fill an entire book. I learned everything you need to know on how NOT to run a multi-million dollar company. Only because I promised myself to give it a try for a year did I stay that long. I was working 100 hours a week, seven days a week; other than time spent with my children, I had no social life. So with quitting came the opportunity to have one.

A friend in Toastmasters was learning to sail a boat so we went out sailing a couple of times. I started going to stock car races, and caught up on the movies. Dancing was something I always thought I would enjoy. I knew nothing about dancing but found a group that met on Saturday nights at the local gym (the owner of the gym was in my Toastmaster group). One Saturday night I showed up by myself to take on ballroom dancing. It was perfect for me, once I understood how it all worked.

The first several times I didn't dance much, because these people knew what they were doing and didn't want to teach me. So what did I do? I found a place that gave ballroom dancing lessons for $5 for 2 hours. Not a bad deal. Then I hooked up with a group that did line dancing because the other challenge I faced was not having a partner. Line dancing solved that problem until I learned ballroom dancing.

As I started to meet people they told me of other dancing going on around Orlando. Within the first month I was dancing four nights a week, with a great 50+ age group crowd, with no drinking or drugs. Even though I was under 50 they let me dance with them.

The only other problem I had was convincing the men that I wouldn't date. I wanted to go home to California, and my fear was that if I met a man I liked I'd get stuck in Florida. So I wouldn't even date.

My self confidence grew and my weight dropped. While dancing I went from a size 24 to a size 4, eating anything I wanted.

By now it was the end of 2000, and I didn't have a job, so to speak, but my living expenses were only $850 per month. Unbelievable but true. I had no credit card debt. My rent was $385 per month, car insurance on my 1993 Toyota Corolla was $50 a month if that, phone & utilities maybe $50, dry cleaning and laundry $50, food and entertainment $200 and my massages $100.

It was time for TJ Seminars to be launched. However, when my partner, who had a wife and child, realized I was serious about taking TJ national, he decided to head down a different path.

All About Solutions was created in TJ Seminars' stead. I started booking seminars on time management, telephone skills, sales training for first time sales people, and consulted with small businesses around Orlando. I was happy, making money and moving forward.

Then I got the bright idea to contact Muzak's competitor, DMX Music, which just so happened to be in Southern California. Go figure how I knew that! I picked up the phone and called the VP of Sales, asking for a personal meeting. My son was getting married in L.A. in March of 2001, and I was given an interview for that time.

To me it was always important to know who your competitors are and what the market is doing. Messages On hold was a product/service that the big guys like Muzak & DMX Music could never develop successfully. I knew the folks at DMX Music were struggling trying to get theirs off the ground.

In our 45 minute meeting, I outlined not one but three different ways we could market On hold Messages for DMX Music. I wanted to do it as a consultant, not as an employee. But one thing lead to another, and they hired me as the sales manager for all of Los Angeles County.

I flew back to Orlando to make the arrangements to move to L.A. in July of 2001, which I did. My new plan was to work for DMX Music for five years, finish this book, live on the beach, and build up my retirement fund. They offered a $100,000 plus salary. I was a happy camper.

I moved in with my mother for a few weeks, while DMX Music was making arrangements for me. To make a long story short, they were going through a corporate change, which included laying off the VP of Sales who hired me. Almost overnight, the entire deal changed to something I wouldn't accept. I left 90 days after I started.

Now I had no job, was renting a room because mom didn't check her HUD housing rules for guests (which meant I couldn't stay with her longer than two weeks), and hadn't been developing All About Solutions for over six months. L.A.'s market is different than Orlando's and with a six months of downtime I should have walked away and gotten a job, but I didn't.

I had no choice but to move in with my children, which was tough, as I tried to sell my seminars. After 60 days I hit the temp agencies and started working for $12 as a receptionist, writing the book, and marketing my seminars at nights and on weekends. By now it was Christmas of 2001

And yes, I started to date. Ended up living with a man in a wheel chair for 4 months while all this craziness was going on. He turned out to be not who he claimed to be, so I moved out.

It was at this time that my stepdaughter, Jennifer, asked me to do a workshop in Stockton, California, which is 80 miles east of San Francisco, and 45 miles south of Sacramento. To anyone in L.A., Stockton was a cow town, and no one I knew lived in Stockton. Jennifer and her husband had just moved to the area and were in love with it. So I took a trip by myself to visit. Jennifer was so insistent that I do a workshop that I told her to "book it". Well she did, and it was an instant success. While on the trip she invited me to move in with them.

In July 2002 I moved by myself to Stockton. Although the seminars were making money, I was writing the book and finding out what it would cost to publish her. To help pay for the book and expenses for running the business, I decided that at nights and on weekends I could work at a retail store.

Macy's gave me a job, and asked where in the store I wanted to work. I figured that since once again I didn't have a social life, I could at least look at the men if I worked in the men's department.

On my second night at work, as a young girl was showing me how to run the cash register, I felt eyes upon me. As I looked up I saw a man who looked like Sean Connery watching me. I smiled, he came over. As he handed me the shirts in his hand, I got nervous and could barely say hello. He paid with a check, which I completely forgot how to process. The little girl (that's how I thought of anyone under 25 years old) showed me how to do it. I apologized to this handsome, sexy looking man in front of me. He came back with "you take as much time as you need, I am perfectly fine!" I turned red and he smiled.

When I got home that night Jennifer asked how my shift went, I told her about this handsome man, but since he didn't ask me out, I figured he was married. I didn't think anything more about it, until a few days later he came back, purchasing more shirts. I was ready and found out he was single, worked as a cabinet maker for 35 years, and also taught at the local junior college for 32 years. But he still didn't ask me out. So now I figured he had a girlfriend. A few nights later he was back, pur- chasing shirts again! Now I find out he has a break from school and has two weeks vacation and no one to go anyplace with. So now I know there is no girlfriend, but he still didn't ask me out.

In the meantime, I was booking seminars and doing them during the day. I landed a seminar in Naples, Florida in August and was excited to go see my sons and their families I had left behind. Because Macy's couldn't get my schedule straight, and the seminars were booking up, I quit and went to Florida for 10 days.

When I returned, my daughter's family was planning a weekend out of town. I had to get back to booking seminars so I stayed behind. At 10 a.m. on Saturday I got a phone call from a friend of my daughter, asking me to go with her and a neighbor to a wine walk fund raiser that night. I didn't want to go but she insisted, so I said "if I get my work done I'll go." At 6 p.m. she came to get Suzie and me.

It was a wonderful August night. Dozens of vendors such as the local markets offered a ton of food to eat, wineries were giving out free wine, there were old classic cars and musicians of all kinds. It was a huge affair.

During the evening an attractive man kept walking by me. On the fifth pass I stepped in front of him and said the classic stupid line, "I know you."

Since I had been in Stockton, I had joined the chamber of commerce, gone to Rotary Club meetings and network meetings and had met dozens and dozens of people. So I really couldn't remember where we had met.

The next thing that came out of my mouth was, "are you Sam? (or George, John, Steve). After each person I named he said "No!" At this point I was totally embarrassed and said, "Okay, before you think I have dated every man in Stockton, what is your name? He was laughing by now and said, "Bob Freeman-Macy's."

We were married on Nov. 7th 2004.

Parenthood

Parenthood

Although I've already written about my sons, I want to tell you a little more about them. Despite all my struggles, and my own history of abuse, I worked hard to give my sons a better life than I'd had. The lives they are living today is the measure of my success.

At 19 years old when I had Alex, no one was there to help me, during the pregnancy or after the delivery. My mother in law, who lived the closest, hated me from the first day she laid eyes on me. My own mother was still with Simon, and not allowed to come and help. I had no idea what to do and finally, after the first two weeks, a woman from the church asked me how I was doing. I burst into tears and she came over a couple of times to help. In 1972 women were still sterilizing everything, and I had no idea how all that worked.

From the beginning Alex was an emotional child; he got that from me, I am sure. When he was just 2 months old I had to go back to work, leaving him in someone's home. Child care then was not what it is today, and then you usually put your child in someone's home. From the beginning he was a problem with baby-sitters, crying all day, and as the years progressed he caused trouble.

Our unstable home life caused most of these problems. Cliff, from whom I was divorced, and I fought all the time. Once Alex went into kindergarten the problems became worse. Plus I was remarried to Dick, who didn't like Alex; I'd had Dave, my third child; and Dick's two children were living with us. Alex was totally rebelling at all of this. On top of all this it was determined that Alex had learning disabilities and his teacher wanted him to repeat kindergarten. I wouldn't agree. The school refused to put him in special education, and by the time kindergarten was over I was exhausted.

First grade was worse than kindergarten because he was totally lost. He had now been tested and 3 of what were eventually determined to be 5 different learning disabilities were discovered; however the principal still refused to put him in special education classes. Alex's behavior was worsening as each week went by. He was large for his age, other children were teasing him, and I was pregnant again with son number four.

Right about the time Alex was in the third grade, after now four years of fighting with the principle to get him into special ed, a friend of mine in the church told me about her fight to get her son extreme special ed; he had brain damage. She taught me so much that at the beginning of the 4th grade when I went into the principal's office insisting Alex get special education, he flatly refused me, and what happened next shocked even me.

I stood up, doubled up my fist, slammed it on his desk, and said, "Fine. Then you will get to meet my attorney," and stormed out. The next week Alex was in special ed!

More testing would show that Alex had been reading the teacher's lips when she read him a story. He had a hearing problem. He would remember the pictures on the page, and when he said he couldn't read, she would read it to him. He would connect the words she said with the pictures. One special ed teacher discovered this when she put her hand over her month and Alex went ballistic.

Alex's emotional behavior was out of control by the time he was 8 or 9 years old. I couldn't leave him alone with his brothers or he would beat on them. One day I came into the living room to find him on top of Dave who was three years old, repeatedly hitting him in the head.

At my wit's end, I called the school; they suggested a child psychologist. Alex and I went to several sessions. At some point in all this they tested his I.Q. which is 139. What the psychologist came up with was that Alex needed to be an only child; I hadn't given him the proper attention as a baby. Jason was just 18 months younger, I went through a divorce when Alex was 3, and remarried when he was 4. Two step children, Ron and Jennifer, came with the new husband; Dave was born the next year, and Don came along two years later, so by the time Alex was 7, I had 6 children to take care of. Given Alex's learning and emotional problems, the psychologist advised that I send him to live with his father, who was still single.

At first I refused; the very thought of sending Alex to live with the man I divorced, and not having him with me, was difficult to comprehend. Cliff loved his children, but he hadn't always done the right thing. I wrestled with this decision for a year, during which Dick would tell me on a regular basis what a bad mother I was for not thinking of my child.

Alex's behavior continued to be out of control. So when he was 10 years old, I sent him to live with his father. I felt like a failure for giving my son away. Even though I had him over on a regular basis, the damage was done. Dave Ziegler talks about the special bond between a mother and a child, and I can attest that it's true. From that day forward Alex felt like I didn't want him, no matter how much I told him I loved him. He felt abandoned.

After high school Alex went to college on a special program for kids with learning disabilities. To our amazement he pulled straight A's! When I asked him how he did that he said, "Every teacher in college just left me alone!"

When he was about 18 I moved to Florida, and didn't offer to take him with me, which he took as another validation to him that I didn't want him around.

At 19 he went on a two year mission for his church, which, with all its rules and regulations, turned out to be as terrible for him as school had been. After that experience he moved to Bakersfield, California and started working for a company trimming trees.

By the time he had worked for this company for about two years, I was calling and talking to him more and more because through my therapy I realized I screwed up with Alex big time.

The guilt I began to experience was becoming difficult to handle. I had learned in therapy to handle situations right away so they don't get out of hand. The situation with Alex was already way out of hand. So I hopped on a plane by myself and flew to Southern California to talk to Alex. We spent a 12 hour day together, driving around Laguna Beach, finding art festivals. Most importantly we talked and talked and talked.

I apologized and apologized and apologized. We cried and cried and cried, after which I said, "I can't change what I did, but now you know why I did it. I can't change how you feel about me. I can't change your childhood. If you never want to talk to or see me again it's totally your choice and I will respect your decision. As for me, I'd love to have you in my life again. My door will always be open to you for the rest of my life." I left wondering what the next day would hold.

A year and a half later Alex moved to Orlando, Florida. One of his dreams was to become a chef (cutting trees was tough work!). Within a month in Orlando he landed a job as a cook.

Alex is now 31 years old, working his way up to sous chef at a 1000 room hotel. He is with a beautiful woman from Ecuador who has two daughters, ages 6 and 11. He calls me every weekend, telling me stories of the girls, his fiance, and how he realizes how tough it is to raise kids.

And, oh yes -- when Bob and I were married, Alex gave me away.

Jason

Jason, son #2, was always a happy-go-lucky kind of child. Everyone he met he talked to and enjoyed. When Alex when to live with his father, Jason assumed the older brother role in our family, and he took the responsibility to heart. I am sure that, going through all that I did while he was a child, I leaned on him, although I tried not to force the care of his brother on him much. At age 13 he was one patch short of becoming an Eagle Scout. He took on leadership roles in our church. Jason always enjoyed a challenge and thrived on being a leader.

We had family meetings on a regular basis to teach the children what to do if there were a fire or an earthquake. Those meetings sure paid off when I was single and working in Hollywood! One morning an earthquake violently shook the ground. This quake happened at 7 a.m., and since I was at work at 6 a.m., I was 20 frightening miles away from my children. For the first 30 minutes I couldn't reach them by phone. The only reason I didn't panic was that I had to get to the boys. Just as I was getting ready to leave work and go home, Jason called me to say that all the boys were fine -- he had done exactly as I taught him to do during a emergency.

Jason was about 14 years old when I divorced Dick. I had married Dick when Alex was 3 and Jason 1, so they grew up with Cliff being their away father and Dick being their at home father. Jason opted to call Dick "Dad." During our nasty divorce Dick turned to Jason one day and said, "You are not my son; I have never loved you."

I will go to my grave never understanding how anyone can hurt a child! Why did he say that?

Given that rejection and my overwhelming stress levels at the time, Jason rebelled and started causing major problems at home. This went on for about six months. Again I had no support from my family, the church members turned on us, and I was backed into a corner. Jason disappeared, or at least I thought he had he was hiding from me. I told him if he did that again he would have to go live with his father. The very next night he did, and that evening I drove him 80 miles to his dad's house, where he stayed for a year or two. After I remarried and moved to Orlando, Florida, Jason called and asked to join me in Florida.

Because I hid the problems in all my marriages from the boys until the divorce came, it was always difficult for them when I would announce yet another divorce. My counselor told me that it was not fair to the boys. But having come from a domestically violent home, living day to day under the thick cloud of stress and depression, I just couldn't bring myself to share my marriage problems with my sons.

Jason loved the social life at school and everyone from students to teachers to janitors knew who Jason was. What surprised the counselors was that Jason hung out with the valedictorians and smart kids, but flunked the 11th grade. At the meeting with the guidance counselor who told me Jason would be held back, I was concerned about him mentally. Flunking a grade in elementary school was one thing but the 11th grade was another, and I was very concerned for my son. As it turned out Jason was perfectly fine with it because he wasn't ready to be an adult.

Although from the age of 14 he had worked and was becoming independent, he needed another year playing in high school. As his friends went on to junior colleges and four year universities, Jason continued working at the hotels which he had done since he was 17 years old. He loved the hotel industry; it seemed to be second nature to him.

Albert, who had worked in the hotel industry for 27 years, had given Jason a summer job as a houseman when he was 17. A houseman delivers towels and sheets to the maids while they are cleaning the rooms. Jason did this for two long hot summers in Orlando. Finally, he moved to the front desk for Albert, then came to work with me in the hotel where I was working, and became a banquet setup person.

From there he became the front desk assistant manager, which turned into the front desk manager shortly after that. Jason continued his upward movement in the hotel industry until at the age of 24 he was the manager a 150 room hotel. At 28 he became the youngest manager of a Hampton Inn in Orlando, the only manager in his company without a college degree, and achieved the largest profit margin of the 13 hotels in his company. At 30, students from Cornell University, which has one of the top hotel management programs in the country, came to review his operations and study why Jason was so successful.

At 26, Jason became the proud father of Carl, and during the worst hurricane season in 50 years of Florida's history 2004, became the proud father of Eddie.

Kate, Jason's wife, is a stay at home mom, so their sons will be well taken care of. Jason is a wonderful father, husband, son and businessman.

Two years ago on Mother's Day, Jason called me. He spent 20 minutes thanking me for the wonderful childhood he had, thanking me for breaking the cycle of abuse in my family, so he could be a great father to Carl. At that moment, whatever trials I had gone through had been worth it, for my son to be the kind of man he is today.

Dave, my third son, was the quietest child in our family. He never cried as a baby unless he was wet or hungry and then you had to listen closely to him, it was more of a whimper than cry. Being the 5th of the children and the 3rd of my children, Dave was pretty much sheltered from what was going on. He was also almost a clone of Dick in his looks and personality. Dave never talked much and analyzed everything.

Dave

Dave was the family jock; at five years old he was in gymnastics and loved it. Just before my divorce from Dick, our money situation improved with my sales job, so we could afford to have a private Olympic-experienced gymnastics coach for him. At 8 or 9 Dave so excelled in gymnastics that he made the team for the California gymnastics competition.

Just prior to the meet, I asked the coach if I should get Dave more training so he would be a contender at the meet; out of 76 positions, Dave had come in 76th. The wise coach told me to let my son be a little boy and enjoy the experience; if Dave wanted to take it to the next level he would do it on his own. The entire family watched as Dave totally enjoyed himself competing and at the end of the day, his final position was something like 45th. Dave would go on to play just about every sport in school, always enjoying the experience.

My concern for him was that he was growing up with a lack of communications skills like his father. So I would make Dave talk to me. When he was younger it was no big deal, but when he got into his teenage years and with the move to Florida without his older brothers, Dave wouldn't talk to anyone. He either played sports or sat in his room.

By this time I had gone through a lot of self-education and knew that communication was always the key to most everything we do. So what I would do with Dave was to go into his room and announce that I was not going to leave until we had a 20 minute talk on any subject he wanted.

The first time I did this, nothing was said for 45 minutes. We both were uncomfortable, but finally he said. "Well, what do we talk about?"

I said, "Anything." We managed to talk about something for 20 minutes. I repeated this everyday for about six months, until we could just talk at anytime and anyplace.

When Dave was 19 and moved out on his own, he got into drugs and the wrong crowd. Orlando is a small town compared to Los Angeles, so I learned through the grapevine what was going on with him.

Word came to me that Dave's roommate, who was dealing in drugs, had a bad drug deal go down in their apartment. The other dealer pulled a gun and pointed it at Dave's face. By the grace of God things went okay, and about 3 days later, while Dave was away from the apartment the Orlando Police Department raided it.

Two days after that Dave stopped by the house, and in our driveway, holding my 19 year old son in my arms, I told him that he and I could do anything together, but I couldn't fix death. I feared for his life if he continued down this path. Within six months Dave had gotten off of drugs and enlisted in the Navy. He traveled all over the world while stationed in Japan, and at the end of his tour, married a beautiful Japanese girl. Now, at 27, he is the father of a two year old baby girl. He works as the accounts receivable manager for a medical supply company in Los Angeles County.

I personally believe that by forcing him to communicate with me when his life was not going well, I could touch his life, and help him see what he was doing.

Don

Don was the youngest of the boys, innocent and trusting from the moment he was born. As a child, he was easygoing, intelligent and analytical, and he is that kind of man today at age 25. He loved school and excelled, even though his brothers teased him about it.

Don was what some people call an old soul; he never was young. I thought it was because being the youngest of four brothers he had to grow up fast to be part of them. But his thoughts were always older thoughts. Once, when he was four years old, he and I were grocery shopping together, I must have been purchasing food for a holiday dinner because the cart was overflowing. As we headed for the checkout counter, he got a serious look on his face and said, "Now, mom, are you sure you have enough money for all this food?"

At 16, Don's older brothers moved back to California to be with their fathers, and he wanted to go also. So I agreed to send him to California to live with his father and stepmother. But I told him I wouldn't interrupt his schooling; he'd have to stay a year. Of course, he begged to come back after only a few weeks, but he stayed the full year and then returned to Florida.

Back home in Orlando, Don's SAT scores were high and he was being offered a scholarship to a local four year college in Orlando. He turned 18 a few months before graduating from high school, and went off the deep end or something. He stopped wanting to go to school, announcing that he was 18 and could do what he wanted. I couldn't figure out what had happened. He lost the scholarship, did finish high school, and took a job at Wolfgang Puck's out at Disney World.

Don got into the drug scene with his brother Dave. In addition, Don drank a lot, so parties, drugs, and alcohol were his life for a few years. One night he almost over-dosed when he took some kind of drugs with alcohol. Some of Don's so-called friends called Alex and Jason (Dave was in Japan at the time) to pick him up. Everyone thought Don was going to die and didn't want him at their house.

I learned later that during the next 24 hours Don went though all kinds of withdrawal and hallucinations from the drugs. The experience was so traumatic for him that from that day forward he hasn't taken another drug.

Now he is in the mortgage financial industry and going to college.

What I think I realized at a young age with the boys is that most likely they would want to experience things in life, whether it was drugs and alcohol or extreme sports. My role was to educate them on the dangers of life and when it was all said and done it would be their choice as to how they lived their lives. Communication with them was the only way I could teach them, because my divorces and marriages didn't really provide good role models for them. However, I was open with them as they became older teenagers and young adults as to my mistakes and why I made them. I explained that no one is perfect, but that asking for forgiveness for our short-comings would speak volumes as to who we are. I taught them to have a conscience and to give everyone they meet in life 100% of themselves.

I told them that I would always love them and be there for them, but that didn't mean I would always sup-port what they did. And above all, I taught them that Our Heavenly Father loved them as well.

How to Begin

The Journey of Self-Empowerment

How to Begin the Journey of Self-Empowerment

As Eleanor Roosevelt has been quoted saying, "No one can make you feel inferior without your permission." Let's take that to the next level: only **YOU** make choices in your life.

If you have gotten to this page, you have already begun. You found the courage and desire to pick up this book and read it. Congratulations! I will tell you that self-empowerment will not come as a gift. You will have to earn it and pay a price to become self-empowered. What does it cost? It's totally up to you. Whether the cost is in dollars, lost relationships, or time, only you can determine whether the price is worth paying. That decision in itself brings self-empowerment.

To begin, there are a few things I need to mention before we start.

First, I am not a psychologist, therapist, or mental health professional. If at any time while reading this book you feel deeply emotional, call a mental health care professional at once! They are trained to help you.

Second, find or develop a support group. It doesn't need to be a formal group; it can be a friend, significant other, sibling, or anyone you know and trust with whom you can talk out your issues. Again, if you are deeply troubled by these topics, seek a mental health care professional.

Third, self-mastery. Bottom line: it's all up to you! No one can help you get to where you want to be but you. NO ONE—therapist, spouse, children, friends, or family—walked every step of the way with me but me. ALL THE EXCUSES STOP RIGHT HERE. Do you want to have a happier, more joyful life? Only you can make it happen.

Fourth, you will move at your own pace—not mine or anyone else's, but yours. Reality is hard to change overnight; too many people try the "quick-fix" method and fail — including me. Through trial and error I learned that making small changes at first built up my self-confidence to tackle larger challenges, which over time, built me a strong foundation from which to stay empowered, even today.

You will need to get out of your comfort zone to make the changes necessary to develop self-empowerment.

Fifth, plan and prepare every step of the way. Don't let life happen to you. That's how you most likely got into the situation you're in. Self-empowerment is taking control of your life by planning. Now does life "happen" while we are doing our plan? You bet, but by having a plan and being prepared, you will be able to handle the situation more easily, more quickly, with more self-confidence, and get back to working your plan.

Sixth, stay teachable. Depending on where you are at in your life and your understanding of human relationships, finances, the opposite sex, career, domestic violence, education, and so many other topics, you need to stay teachable, because you are going on a learning curve like no other.

For example, if your goal is to become an attorney like Francine Ward, who went from hooker to attorney, then you will need to figure out how to get through college. I don't know about you, but I long ago gave up the idea that I had a rich relative someplace. Now, you must become an expert on student loans, grants and scholarships, not to mention choosing which college to attend.

Seventh, through this process be gentle with yourself by giving yourself rest and rejoice time. It may be an hour, a month, or even a year, but realize what you are about to go through is difficult. Rest and rejoice often.

The Paralysis
of Fear

The Paralysis of Fear

For many years, fear was my best friend, because we had been together for so long. Mastering this learned emotion will set you free for the rest of your life. Care must be taken that in your zeal to heal you don't move backwards. This took me the longest to understand and control, because up until then this emotion had governed my entire life.

There are two ways we experience fear- internal and external. Simply put, internal fear is all those thoughts that are inside our head. External fear is visible. They do work together in a good way if we have proper balance. Let's say you are walking in the woods and see what you think is a snake. At first your eyes tell you it's a snake and to run the other way; external. However, your brain tells you to stop and take a closer look; it's a stick; internal. The nature of trauma is "not in the external event but in the internal meaning and experiences of the event" (Ziegler, 2001).

To illustrate, the most paralyzing fear I had to overcome was tall men. Max was five times larger than I was; as a result I felt frightened when a large man came near me. I literally froze and couldn't speak. Internally, I felt that this large man would hurt me.

The way I finally overcame this fear was by becoming the first woman in a previously all-male Toastmasters club. At the time, I didn't realize I was overcoming this fear; I just wanted to learn how to speak in public. For the first six weeks, every Friday when we held our meetings, I got physically sick when I walked into the room. I would repeatedly tell myself that none of these men was going to hurt me. Then I would introduce myself to a few of the members each week, asking questions about who they were, their personal and business lives, hobbies and so on. I would replace old memories of men abusing me with new memories of wonderful, kind, caring, giving men, who supported me with my goals and desires in business. This process took me six weeks; once I got through meeting all the men I no longer became physically sick. In fact, just short of two years after I joined, they elected me president of the club.

Self-Mastery

Self-Mastery

This is the heart of *A Wallflower No More*. If you decide to take on the challenges of changing your life forever, the next several pages will provide for you the ability to build a solid foundation of self-mastery so self-empowerment can develop. You will be able to direct, manage, and create your own life. It won't be easy. You will become frustrated with yourself, your friends, your family, co-workers, the "system," and will wonder from time to time if this has all been worth it.

As Anthony Robbins says in *Notes from a Friend*, "If you look at any of the most successful people in history, you will find this common thread: They would not be denied. They would not accept "no." They would not allow anything to stop them from making their vision, their goal, a reality" (Robbins, 1995).

I am here to tell you with every fiber of my being, IT IS WORTH IT! It's worth getting rid of the preprogrammed voices in your head that haunt you night and day. It's worth the struggle to "know" where you are going in life, not just wonder. It's worth it when you start to see people treat you the way you desire to be treated. It was worth it when I broke the cycle of abuse in my family. Tears of joy streamed down my face as my son, holding his newborn son in his arms said, "Thanks, Mom." It doesn't get any better than this! So yes, it's worth it all!

So what is the definition of self-mastery? Self is you... Mastery, by Webster's definition, is: victory in struggle. You are building a foundation of self-mastery to develop self-empowerment. In other words, self-mastery is a series of victories over your individual demons to build a good foundation of self-empowerment.

Changing years of bad habits and replacing them with empowering habits may not come easy. In the remainder of the pages of this chapter, I am going to cover areas in my life that I felt I needed to be changed, improved, or understood—personal growth and development, human relations, and finances—that would lead me to self-mastery. The purpose of these topics is to give you a solid foundation to build self-mastery, which will lead to self-empowerment.

Guideline #1

Set your goals to fit the real situation. Take baby steps instead of trying to get right to the finish line first. From birth, I have always been competitive, so starting out slow and easy was very difficult for me. I always wanted to be first. Self-mastery is not being competitive with anyone but you. The entire point of setting realistic goals is to learn to become successful at what you set out to do, thereby replacing negative thoughts about yourself with positive ones.

A woman I know felt out of control with her weight, her smoking and her job. She decided on the weekend that the following week, she was going to start a diet, stop smoking, and start her new job. On top of all that, she was scheduled to have a minor surgery. After listening to her frustration, my question to her was, "Why are you setting yourself up to fail?" Like my friend, the pain of where we are is so great that we want to fix it all in one week. I know I tried that way and I failed. Self-empowerment comes with baby steps.

Guideline #2

Make a realistic list of where you are presently in each of the areas listed above and act accordingly. For example, if you can't make this month's rent, finding a second job to pay the rent is more important than enrolling in college.

Maintaining daily survival while planning for the future was real for me because there was no other way to move forward. Sound difficult? Well, it was. But I did it and so can you.

Guideline #3

Reward yourself often, learn to love the unique person that you are, and realize that every baby step you take moves you towards self-empowerment and is a victory over your past. As I started down this difficult path of self-empowerment, I needed encouragement. So I enacted a reward system for myself to give me the encouragement I needed to continue.

The rewards ranged from flying from Florida to Washington State to meet my step-brothers, to specialty coffee, to clothes, to movies, to dinner with friends. Cost doesn't matter; the reward you chose should mean something to you.

Guideline #4

Books and audio tapes were the medium from which I chose to learn. They were free at the library. I was such a frequent borrower that the librarians knew me by name. As my financial situation improved, I purchased them, so they would be there to reread or listen to at any time. In fact, my books and tapes were so important to me that when I moved back to California from Florida, I left the dishes, towels, and other household things to bring my books and tapes with me.

Remember the story of Abraham Lincoln, who read everything he could get his hands on. He would walk miles and miles to get a book. Read, and never stop reading and/or learning, it's the only way you can get from where you are to where you want to be.

In the reference section of this book, you will find pages of books and audio tapes that were and still are my best friends.

Financial

Financial problems are what led me into two bad marriages. I figured Cliff, my first husband, and I could work together as a team. Little did I know that he didn't want to work at all! Still feeling invisible, I left that marriage without a job. Struggling with the two boys, I married Dick, my second husband, for financial security. He had been at his job for eight years.

I was in my late twenties when I started realizing that the need to plan my financial future was a must. When I made the decision to divorce for the second time, unlike my first divorce, I had four children to worry about. I had been working for two years in sales, making good money, so I felt financially secure.

Since then I have planned and calculated every aspect of my financial world. Divorcing for the third time left me in a positive financial state to move back to California. Have I always been right? No. What I learned was not to make the same mistakes over and over.

Later on in the book, I will talk about basic financial planning to surviving while you are getting educated to become even more financially sound.

A Gentle Thunder

For Jayne

*A gentle thunder fills the air, as the waves of the ocean
crash around you.*

*Giving you the strength to burn those fields of sadness
within.*

*By Aurora Ashton
May 16, 2002*

Personal Growth & Development

Define Yourself
Never be content with someone else's definition of
YOU!
Instead, define YOURSELF by
Your own beliefs,
Your own truths,
Your own understanding of who you are and
How you came to be.
AND NEVER BE CONTENT UNTIL YOU ARE
HAPPY
WITH THE UNIQUE PERSON YOU ARE!

Author Unknown

What you are about to embark on is the discovery of who you are! This concept is as simple as that. For me, this journey of personal growth was difficult and long, mostly because when I started my journey, I was 39 years old. I would give you a middle-of-the-road answer to any question, because I didn't want to offend anyone. I didn't want to make waves, so I took the wallflower approach, trying to be invisible.

Who are you? was the question I would ask when I was teaching telephone techniques, time management, and organizational skills. Many of us, somewhere along the way, have forgotten who we are deep inside. Answering the following questions will help you start your journey to self-empowerment.

1. Do you like to get up at 4:00 a.m. or sleep until noon?
2. Do you like to be indoors or outdoors?
3. Do you like hard physical activities or lighter ones?
4. Do you prefer to read or watch TV?
5. Are you competitive or passive?
6. Do you like theater, ballet, or opera?
7. What type of music do you enjoy?
8. Do you like cold or hot weather?
9. Do you like children? Seniors? Young adults?
10. What type of movies do you watch?

This list could go on forever. It important to find out who you are and what your likes and dislikes are.

One day, at a business chamber mixer, a man asked me this question: "What does Jayne like to do in her spare time?" It stopped me cold! "What spare time?" was my response! That little question depressed me because I didn't know who Jayne was. I went home that night and started the above list, which was much longer, then went onto another list that showed me where my life was headed at the time.

I was 39 and married but sleeping in a separate bedroom from my husband, with 3 teenage boys at home. I was living in Orlando, Florida, in debt, weighing 205 pounds, with intense back pain, no college education, no real friends, and no clue where I was going or how to get there. I was scared as hell!

I made a list of areas in my life that I thought I needed to change and improve.

1. Develop hobbies.
2. Gain an education.
3. Improve my marriage.
4. Exercise.
5. Diet.
6. Spend time with my sons.
7. Extend family responsibilities.
10. Find a job.
11. Make friends.
12. Stay informed by reading and watching the news.
13. Continue my healing process.
14. Write in my journal.
15. Improve my personal appearance.
16. Learn manners and proper etiquette.

The list was over five pages; as it grew I became even more depressed. How in the world was I going to overcome, change and progress with such a long hard difficult list? After a couple weeks, I started to use the prioritizing skills I'd learned from working in sales. It's simple: list every area in your life you want to change or improve, then place them in order of importance. Prioritizing is a tool that will serve you well as you take this journey. My five-page list was too much to handle, so I had to fit the items into one of the eight categories below. My list now looked something like this:

1. Self-esteem
2. Personal growth and development
3. Family
4. Financial
5. Emotional & mental wellness
6. Human relations
7. Diet/exercise
8. Career

Now this list was manageable.

I worked on each area, as it became important in my life. While working your way through this list, you'll find out many things about yourself. For instance, one great discovery I made was that I hate meatloaf! I always made it and ate it, because it was easy on the budget. Here is how it empowered me to know that. My husband loves meatloaf. Now, if I stood back and said, "I don't like it so I won't cook it for you," how selfish would that be? I choose to cook it for him and make something else for myself.

Self-Esteem

One of the first areas on which I worked was self-esteem. Why? Because if I didn't believe in myself, I couldn't complete the process to self-empowerment.

Webster defines self-esteem as: Belief in oneself; self-respect. Self-esteem is the core to self-empowerment. I read, years earlier, that if all you ever teach your children was good self-esteem, the rest will follow. How interesting that I worked for years building my sons' self-esteem but didn't think to work on my own. I didn't feel worthy of such standards. "You are stupid, ugly and no man will want to marry you." Simon told me that for over 10 years. Women and children in environments of domestic violence start believing what their abusers say to them.

So for me to start developing higher self-esteem, I had to deal with the old belief that I was stupid, and prove to myself otherwise.

Because Simon said I was stupid, I believed I had a learning disability. My belief was based on two factors: 1) My oldest son had a learning disability; 2) for over 20 years, I enrolled in college every September; by each October, I had dropped out. For me, this all confirmed what he had said every day. It didn't matter that I didn't have support from a husband; it didn't matter that I was working 70 hours a week; it didn't matter that I was raising six children. It never dawned on me that those things could have been the reasons I dropped out of college each year.

"You are stupid" rang in my head for over 20 years. Now it was time to FIND OUT if it was true. Although I had a high school diploma, I received special permission to enroll in the GED program at the local high school, and I requested to be tested for learning disabilities.

When the results came in, I didn't believe the results because they didn't go along with what the voice in my head was saying: "You're stupid!" The people at the high school obviously didn't know what they were doing. So, I went to the local junior college and requested to be tested again.

An elderly woman at the junior college came in to give me the test results. My initial thought was, "Oh my goodness, it's worse than I thought. They sent a grandmother to tell me the bad news!"

Here is what she said: "You don't have learning disabilities. We have determined that what you had was a traumatic childhood with abuse going on daily. The way we know this is that your education is spotted. You can multiply fractions, but you can't add them."

As I walked out of her office, my self-esteem raised 10 levels. I had taken a major step to empower myself. I had disproved something that I had believed in all my life. I was not stupid!

Analyze to Change

Most of you knew I'd come to the subject of "change" sooner or later. When I say this word, you instantly hear groans and grumblings. Why? Because we are creatures of habit, who like to stay in our "comfort zone." When you demand for someone to get out of his or her "comfort zone," you will get resistance. I was no different; when I reviewed my list of things I should change about myself, it was overwhelming. In fact, it was at this stage that I almost gave up. There was too much to change, and I didn't know how to go about it.

As I contemplated what to do, whether to give up or change, I remembered where I had come from and what had been taken from me. That old determined spirit kicked in and I decided to jump in with both feet. I certainly wasn't happy with where I had come from, the future looked more promising than the past. It was at this crossroads that I decided to NEVER give up or go back. So the only way was to move forward and that meant I had to CHANGE!

Where to start was the next question. So I analyzed where my time was going each day. Seven hours sleeping, two hours driving the kids to school, sports, etc., nine hours working (which included an hour for lunch), a half-hour computing, two hours cooking, cleaning, washing clothes, shopping, three-and-a-half hours watching television. There is where my 24 hours a day were spent.

Immediately you see the three-and-a-half hours of watching television, which was an area I could eliminate and spend working on my list. However, as I started to use that time for myself, Albert insisted that I sit with him to watch television. Since one of the items on the list was to improve our relationship, I did as he requested.

So, while watching the twentieth rerun of his favorite sitcoms, I read books on self-development. While driving the kids around town, I would share my newfound knowledge with them. They were my audience, trapped because they needed the ride. I used other times to my advantage. For example, I would use my lunch hour to go to the library or dry cleaners or whatever else needed to be done. Little by little, I squeezed out time for my personal development. I was building stronger relationships with the boys, and finding out who Jayne really was, all at the same time.

The point is this: analyze every minute in your day, adjust and readjust your time until you are doing those things that help build your foundation of self-empowerment.

Review your list daily or weekly, because your priorities will change depending on what your focus is and what is currently happening in your world that day.

Controlling Emotions by Understanding the Brain

Emotions can govern your life, if you let them. Understanding how the brain works will help you when you find yourself in those highly emotional situations.

"Because the brain develops around experience, early influences can have lifelong impact, with trauma increasing the likelihood of stress-related psychiatric disorders" (Ziegler, 2002).

For instance, did you know that most of us cannot use the emotional side of our brain and the logical side at the same time? What's the importance of this little tidbit of knowledge? When you find yourself in an emotional situation, in order to handle it rationally, start by making a list of the positives and negatives. This forces your brain to move from emotion to logic, thereby giving you the physical ability to calm down during a crisis!

Bringing It All Together

Once I analyzed all of the above, I was ready to move forward. I took on each separate area on the list. I reviewed it for its importance in my life, how much I needed to change, and where I wanted to be when I was finished. I used the old saying, "If you don't know where you're going, you won't know when you get there." I understood that many of these areas would be forever evolving and changing. Believe it or not, change is good.

A perfect example is my love for football. From age 6 to 49, I loved football. I could talk about the players, the coaches and the teams. On our first date, my present husband took me to a golf course to see if I would like golf. After a 15-minute lesson, I hit my first ball 10 yards! I was hooked; football is now second to golf in my life. The willingness to change and explore new worlds has led me to a newfound passion: golf.

I have come to learn that it's through change that we continue to evolve in our lives, have new experiences and make new friendships, and stay mentally young.

Physical Well-being

It hasn't been that long since scientists didn't fully understand that there was a connection between our bodies, mind, and spirit. The leap in scientific studies in this area during the last several years has been unbelievable. Why is this important to you? If you are recovering from an abusive environment, the understanding of how the mind, body, and spirit work together to make you who you are is vital to your recovery; it's necessary to heal all three.

When Jennifer, my stepdaughter, was going through school to become a massage therapist, she learned that if your body was beaten at anytime in your life, that exact spot on your body will remember and REACT to any physical touch in that area.

How does that help you on this journey to self-empowerment? If you know why you react to a situation ahead of time, you can overcome, reverse and heal from what has happened to you.

Remember, I was 6 years old when Max placed his large hands around my neck and squeezed the breath out of me.... From that day forward, if anyone touched my neck I stopped breathing and froze. My brain would be telling me that my female friend who reached over and touched my necklace wasn't Max, but my body's memory took over and reacted to the memory of this powerful event.

To heal from these memories, I started to massage my own neck, telling myself that no one was going to hurt me. Old memories of fear and pain were replaced with new memories of love and nurturing. Now when my husband touches me, I respond with love, not fear.

Self-induced abuse is common among sexually abused children. Many children hate their bodies for responding to intercourse or fondling. Our bodies did not know we were children; our bodies respond naturally. Many people choose to punish their bodies by cutting, scalding, or mutilating themselves.

Other methods of self-induced abuse are drugs, alcohol, and food. How blessed I was that neither drugs nor alcohol were ever an issue with me. They could have been; when I was 16, dressing in the high school locker room, a girl came up to me held out her hand with some very colorful pills and said, "Go ahead, take them." At that instant a voice inside my head said, "If you take those pills, you will hurt your unborn children." That voice was so loud and clear that I turned around to see who else was there. We were alone; once again, my Heavenly Father guided me.

What's important to know is that back in 1969 it was not commonly known that drugs could stay in your body for years and cause birth defects to a fetus.

Love Your Body

Instead of turning to drugs or alcohol, I would eat for comfort. My pattern of overeating was what sent me over 205 pounds by the time I was done going through intense therapy!

On the flip side, there are the many people who have been abused who have gone the other way, becoming anorexic, hating their bodies so much that they starve themselves to death. The mindset for people like this is control of their bodies. Professional counseling is recommended for both of these types of eating disorders.

When I weighed 205 pounds, a cute little young girl who had just finished her B.S. in nutrition came to our Toastmaster group (other women joined after I did) and talked on nutrition and weight. At the conclusion of her talk, she reached down and from under the podium pulled out a five-pound piece of fat. The gasp from the entire audience came at once as she said, "This is only five pounds of the fat you are carrying in your body."

Now I am going to try and walk very softly here and try to make myself very clear. No matter what your weight is, 90 or 205, you love yourself for who you are, not how you look. At 205 pounds, I tried almost every diet you could think of, but the weight stayed with me. I remember standing in front of the mirror one day, saying to myself, "I love you no matter how much you weigh." It was shortly after the acceptance of my body that I found a diet and exercise program that worked for me.

When I went from a size 24 to a size 4, my doctor told me to quit trying to lose weight. He said, "Women just think they need to be thin." He had been our family doctor for 11 years. I laughed. Two years earlier he had accused me of cheating on the diet he had put me on. I said, "Look at your chart. I weigh 140, and wear a size 4. Now tell me what the charts say I should weigh for my height and age." His eyes got big and he said, "Well, I don't care what the charts say. Don't lose any more weight." My next comment was, "Don't worry, I will never have a problem with being too thin, because I love food too much and struggle each day to stay where I am."

This is a good lead-in to the subjects of diet and exercise. There are hundreds of diet plans, however I don't believe in being on a diet. I do believe that diet plans are the vehicle you need to change your eating habits. If your eating habits don't change, you will always be overweight.

Make no mistake about it, I love food, I enjoy food, and food makes me feel good. However, food was slowly killing me. National studies are constantly telling us how dangerous being overweight can be to your health. "A new study from HHS' Centers for Disease Control and Prevention (CDC) that shows poor diet and inactivity are poised to become the leading preventable cause of death among Americans—causing an estimated 400,000 deaths in 2000. CDC estimates that 64 percent of all Americans are overweight, including more than 30 percent who are considered obese." (FDA).

Watch and listen to what your body is telling you. I went on a high-protein diet to lose 70 pounds. However, once I started introducing all the food groups back into my diet, I started gaining weight. Understanding portion control was the next thing I had to learn about keeping the weight off.

If you have 10 pounds or more to lose, my heart goes out to you. If you stay honest with yourself, focus on your goals, and reward yourself often, you can lose weight. Self-mastery over food has led to self-empowerment to control my weight. Don't go on a diet! Change your eating habits, instead; you are guaranteed to keep the weight off.

Exercise

Exercise is an activity I never enjoy. As a result of the car accident I have no choice but to exercise. I do have a choice to exercise my way. Being in a gym isn't for me, nor is running 10 miles a day. I have to lift a few weights to maintain my skeleton; this keeps me from being in intense pain. Walking and bicycling give me an intense cardiovascular workout, which is important for good health. I have learned over the last 10 years that if you design your own fitness plan with the help of a fitness expert, you'll be more likely to stick with it.

In addition to exercising like walking, running, biking and weight lifting, stretching is a great way to stay limber

Last fall my back went into muscle spasms so bad that I was walking sideways, hurting beyond belief with every step. After a couple of days of this I decided to go to the doctor, thinking he would give me the usual anti-inflammatory drugs and tell me to stay in bed. He gave me the drugs but showed me how to do simple stretching exercises to stop the muscle spasms and strengthen my back. He promised me that if I did these simple stretching exercises each day I would never have muscle spasms.

I took his bet because the pain was so intense I feared the pain more than the stretching. Each day I stretched before I even got a cup of coffee. Four months after that, while I was out playing golf, I hit the ground with my club, and instantly my back went into spasms. After taking 5 minutes to regain my composure, I walked over to a bench and did my stretching. The spasms stopped and I played the next hole without pain. A friend with whom we play golf said he has never found anything easier than stretching that gives you such a high rate of return for your efforts.

Go to the library or book store and pick up a book on stretching exercises; they will do you a world of good.

It's another proven fact that the older you get, the more you need to exercise to maintain a healthy life. So get over it like I did and find out what is best for you, your body, and your lifestyle. You will feel better, have more energy, and build up your self-esteem along the way. Not a bad return for just 15-20 minutes a day.

If you are on drugs, alcohol, or have any other behavior patterns going on that are hurting you, seek out a professional counselor today! Please!

Human Relations

Unless you decide to become a monk so you don't have to interact with other people, this section on human relations development will become invaluable to you.

To me, the definition of human relations is my relationship to everyone else. This, I realized, takes knowing who I am before I can know who the other person is.

Whether it is family, friends, co-workers, or strangers on the street, how I relate to each one of these people is important to my daily life.

Personality types should be taught in high school, college and for anyone who has to work with others. Another way of looking at this knowledge is learning to "read" people. Now, most likely if you are over 50 years old and never read a book on personality types, you can "read" people just because in 50 years you came across all types of people. If you were in a box most of your life, like I was, this lack of knowledge led me into a couple of bad relationships, jobs, and other difficult situations in my life.

There are basically four personality types: analytical, driver, amiable and expressive. It's important to first find out who you are so you can learn how the other personalities affect you and you affect them. Here is a basic outline of each personality type:

Analytical: is a fact person, goes by the numbers.

Driver: wants it done now, doesn't want to hear why it's not done.

Amiable: is the "OK, that's fine" person, very easygoing.

Expressive: is the office clown, wants to make everyone laugh.

It's important to understand that there are no right or wrong personality types, they just are! You can be one or several of these types depending on your environment. At home you could be expressive, but at work analytical.

Doctors Robert Bolton and Dorothy Grover Bolton have done extensive research on this subject; in their book, *People Styles at Work (1996)*, they reviewed 16 personality types. That was way over my head, so I stuck to the basic four. Once you learn the other types, you can communicate with those people more effectively, thereby making life easier for you.

Learning about personality types changed my life. Once I realize which personality I was, other people became easier for me to understand.

A perfect example is Sally, a close friend of mine for over 17 years. Sally called me almost daily to give me a blow-by-blow of her life with an alcoholic husband. For years, I listened and sympathized with her. Twice, I let her and her daughters stay with my family for a week while he was on a drunken rampage. She always went back and became the martyr.

What really hit home with me is when Sally sabotaged his recovery. Within two months, the cycle started again. It was then that I realized she was drawing energy from me but wasn't going to change.

On my journey of self-empowerment, I realized I had to leave our draining relationship. I couldn't control Sally; I could only control my life by making the decision to end this relationship.

As you go, weigh each of your personal and professional relationships; be honest with yourself. Is it healthy for both of you? Ask yourself: Do I feel empowered and positive, or do I feel negative and angry? When I leave this person are my energy levels drained or overflowing?

Self-empowerment comes from having strong healthy relationships with the people around you. By being honest in your evaluation of each of these relationships you empower yourself. When you interact with these people, whether you set limits with the driver personality at work by stating the time-frame in which you will get your part of his project done or have to pull information out of an amiable family member, you will know what to say, how to say it, and when to say it. And that, my friend, is self-empowerment.

The Magic of Mentors

One of the fastest ways to advance your career is by using mentors. Without my realizing it at the time, my first mentor assigned herself to me when I worked at the Cally Curtis Co. She gave me all the tools I needed to become successful as a novicesales person.

Later, while in a seminar, the instructor said something about finding a mentor to speed your career along, gain knowledge, and avoid common mistakes or pitfalls. It was than that I realized how much my sales manager at Cally Curtis had helped me.

Through the years I have had several mentors, some lasting one day, others lasting 5 years. Here are a few characteristics you should look for when choosing a mentor.

Mentor Characteristics

1. Many years of experience in your area or field of interest.
2. Willingness to share their knowledge.
3. The time to be a mentor.
4. Core values that match your own.
5. Male vs Female -- it doesn't matter; just make sure that if this person is of the opposite sex they and you are clear on the business goals.
6. Are they in your company or outside? 99% of the time I chose outside my company.
7. You need to trust them. What they are going to tell you may not be what you want to hear but they are the expert and you should be able to trust them .
8. Communicate on an ongoing basis .

Mentee Characteristics

1. Be teachable .
2. Be honest.
3. Analyze what they are telling you. The decisions will ultimately be yours.
4. Communicate.
5. Be ready to get out of your comfort zone and learn.
6. Don't abuse the situation by calling your mentor every hour of the day. Set down a clear pattern for communication.

7. Outline what it is you need from your mentor.
8. Saying thank you a lot goes a long way.
9. If you and your mentor are not jelling than change mentors

At first I didn't understand that there are people out there who love to share their knowledge and experience. Now I totally understand that giving back is how we empower ourselves and move forward. The pride that you have when you see someone you care about moving forward in your life is a lot like raising children. It doesn't get better than that.

Don't feel this should just be for a career. Mentors can be useful in your personal life as well. When my older son had learning disabilities another woman in the church sat me down and explained how the school system worked and what the laws of California said regarding educating children. Armed with this information, I obtained special education for Alex.

Emotional/Mental Wellness

Emotional/mental wellness is a very involved topic. My suggestion is to gather books and read all you can on the subject. In *Stress for Success (1998)*, James Loehr explains that emotions do run your life, and you can control them. It's an awesome book.

One very important lesson Ann taught me in therapy was how to deal with others who were trying to emotionally control me. What I learned from my abusers was that by emotionally controlling everything and everyone around me, as they did, I had power. That's not true. What is true is that you can only control yourself.

By understanding this principle, I also learned that I was responsible for my own mental and emotional wellness. If I am being attacked verbally, only I can stop it, by asking the attacker to stop or by removing myself from the situation. I cannot control what another person does, says, or thinks. Self-empowerment comes from understanding that I can only control myself.

Affirmations

A key element in my moving forward with self-empowerment was replacing the old records playing inside my head. "You are stupid" was the hardest to overcome because the deep seated planting that was done. After I found out I didn't have learning disabilities I had to set down a way to overcome those voices.

Affirmations were the tools I used to accomplish this goal. I read someplace that it takes seven positives to counter one negative. What a depressing ratio but nonetheless there it was so I designed a plan. In my opinion, sticky notes are the greatest invention of the last century. Choosing bright colored sticky notes, I wrote affirmations like these:

- You are smart.
- You can do anything you put your mind to.
- If it is to be it ís up to me.

I placed these notes and many, many others all over the house, the car and my office and repeated them to myself dozens of times a day. The last one above is a key affirmation because it brings the responsibility back to me which is where it belongs.

As an adult I was and am responsible for all that happens in my life. Before, I would let the school counselor or my husband or some salesperson tell me what to do -- whether it was to send my son to live with his father, do all the work around the house, or purchase a $7,000 dollar solar unit. In all those cases it was my responsibility to learn or find out what the situation was and what the outcome of those decisions would be.

Within days of reading and re-reading these affirmations strange new feelings started welling up inside of me. At work, if asked to take on a major project that no one else wanted, I would boldly stand up and say, "I'll do it." Six months later when the apartment industry took hold for our company, the other five sales people wanted to jump on board to reap the rewards. Being a sharing person I trained them all; the result was my promotion to national sales manager.

Start with one affirmation or a dozen -- it doesn't matter. What happens inside your brain when you read and re-read affirmations is that the subconscious takes over. Many believe the subconscious is like a computer whose job it is to solve problems and validate what's been put into it.

Example: If for years you have said "you are stupid" the subconscious believes what it's told. Now when it's time to take a college entrance exam the subconscious steps up and repeats what your (or someone you believed was telling you the truth) told it. As you get out of your car headed for the building, your subconscious says, "Why are you doing this? You are stupid." Walking up to the room where the exam will take place your subconscious grabs your stomach and loudly says, "Stop, why are you doing this? You are stupid." As you find a seat, your subconscious, getting really upset yells, "Who do you think you are? You are stupid." Five minutes before the test begins your subconscious tells your body that you're in danger and all kinds of body functions start to take place: sweating, nausea, light headedness, and then the bowels kick in, so you run to the bathroom where your subconscious really gets serious. "You will fail at this. You are nobody, you are nothing, you have tried this before and lost. Now go home and remember that you are stupid."

Affirmations play a huge role in countering the subconscious. By replacing those negative thoughts with something like "Someone told me I was stupid, but let's find out for sure. Who do I think I am? I am Jayne and will stop at nothing to become self-empowered. If I fail, at least I tried. If it is to be it's up to me, regardless of the outcome" you can literally change the course of your life.

Money
Management

Financial Survival

When Columbus and his explorers first set foot in the Americas, the natives were using seashells as a monetary unit. The best known form of money among the Native Americans north of Mexico was wampum. It was made out of the clamshells.

As the Pilgrims began settling in the new land, they lived in communes, where everyone worked and benefitted equally from the fruits of each other's labor. This was the most efficient means of survival in a harsh and difficult setting; more could be achieved as a group than as individuals. As shiploads of new people arrived, communities became townships, townships became cities, and continental society changed to meet the needs of this ever growing and changing group of people.

A shoemaker learned that if he made an extra pair of shoes, he could barter for life staples, such as eggs and milk. A country of entrepreneurs was born. If you worked very hard, you could get what you needed and wanted.

Why the history on money? Because money, and the understanding of how to use it, is extremely important to self-empowerment. It's vital to learn how to make it, manage it and save it. Money is your ticket to independence.

The Millionaire Next Door (1996), by Thomas J. Stanley, Ph.D., and William D. Danko, Ph.D., is an outstanding book for you to read. When you learn how wealthy Americans became that way, it will surprise you. Three quick examples: most millionaires do not own a suit, drive an expensive car or make over $100,000 a year. What they do or did was manage their money over time.

As you will see, money management is the key to financial survival. It doesn't matter how much money you make, it's how you spend and save it that will lead you to self-empowerment.

Money: Making It

Figuring out how much you make is simple. **Gross** is what you make before taxes and other deductions. **Net** is what you bring home. There are other ways to have income: child support, alimony, interest on savings accounts, and investments. The important thing here is if you have any of these other income sources, make sure they are reliable from month to month.

Managing It

Now, herein lies the hard part. Money is more than elusive... it's slippery. Ever go to the movies, drop $100 and not realize it? Think FRUGAL. Did you know that most millionaires in our country never received a dime of inheritance nor had their college paid for by someone else? What they did do was manage all aspects of their financial situation.

Spending It

As you are putting a personal budget together, you may believe that your expenses are endless. However, in reality, you only have four recurring expenses for survival: food, shelter, clothing, and utilities.

Additionally, the list of things you spend your money on could include the following: childcare, car payment and maintenance, cell phone, cable TV, attorney fees, savings account, car insurance, credit card debt, health insurance, medical bills, education expenses, personal loans, gifts, entertainment. This list could be endless. Again, you really only have four basic recurring survival expenses to be concerned about.

However, before I talk about those four basic expenses, what should be mentioned is the definition of *needs* and *wants*. Simply put, needs are things or items you must have daily to survive. Wants are everything else. That is why the needs list is so short: food, shelter, clothing and utilities. You need those four things or items to survive. Let's start with shelter.

Shelter

Housing is usually your largest expense each month. When considering housing, consider whether the location is convenient to your job, schools, childcare, bus systems, grocery stores, etc. First and foremost, it should be in a safe place. It may take longer to find, but if you look hard enough, you can find affordable housing in a safe area. Check with the police department; they will tell you what the crime rate is in your area.

For example, my daughter-in-law in Florida shopped apartment rents and found a large apartment in a better area for $200 a month less than her current rent. Make some phone calls; do yourself a favor and research! It could save you a bundle.

When purchasing a home, get all the facts first. Prices vary among states and areas within a state. California, for example, is much more expensive than Florida.

You'll need to consider the down payment, the property taxes, home repairs, and all of the other expenses. Figure all these things in. If you can purchase a home in a good area, with the idea of living there for a few years, then do it. Equity in a home will bring you wonderful benefits in the future.

Food

Food is an area where you can be flexible with money without sacrificing nutrition. It does take time, planning, and work. Fast food is no substitute for home-cooked, nutritious food. It's expensive, and it isn't good for you. You can make meals ahead of time for weekdays, then refrigerate or freeze them so they are readily available.

Managing your food budget starts with meal planning. What are you going to eat this week? If you are a cooking whiz, this won't be a problem for you. I had to get help from cookbooks. I started with an easy-to-follow one.

When planning the week's meals, use leftovers in other dishes. For example, a roast can be used to make sandwiches, stews, soups, tacos, and as a topping for salads. Potatoes, once cooked, can be added to soups and stews. Mashed potatoes can be flattened like a pancake and fried in olive oil for dinner.

In other words, don't toss it out until you've thought of all the ways you can use it. Old bread (though not moldy) can be used to make croutons, stuffing, and bread pudding. Older tomatoes can be used in sauces, marinara, spaghetti and tacos. Hard grated cheese can be put in omelets.

Also, know how food is sold in the store. A bag of potatoes is cheaper than individual potatoes. Purchase the bag and make multiple meals from it.

Make a list of everything you need at the store, and don't leave anything out. BUT DO NOT ADD to this list while shopping. Remember, you are on a budget. Impulse buying can quickly increase your food expenditures.

Clip coupons for only those items you want to purchase. A coupon for something you don't need is NOT a savings. Give it to someone else. When I had an army to feed three times a day, I was a member of a "coupon club." We would mail each other coupons that we didn't want and request ones we wanted.

I also belonged to a food co-op. Since we lived 30 miles from downtown Los Angeles, where there was a food distribution market, a group of 40 women got together and determined that we could save money and get better quality food by making the trip to L.A. twice a month. We each used our talents and resources to benefit the co-op. One woman had a huge garage; I utilized my organization talents to arrange the garage for the distribution of the food. Two women drove huge vans; they did the shopping. Yet another woman loved finances and kept our books. I participated for three years and saved an average of $200 per month.

Most families will eat the same thing once each week, or at least once each month. This is a key piece of knowledge, because it will save you money. You can purchase these items on sale and in bulk knowing you'll use them.

If there is no access to a food co-op in your area, it's important that you become very well acquainted with at least three grocery stores nearby. You should familiarize yourself with all of the items in each store that your family eats. What do these items cost, on average? When do they go on sale? Do a cost comparison between each store. If the cost difference isn't more than 5%, only go to one store. Usually, you will make up the difference on another item. Gasoline is expensive, and you could spend that 5% in gas just getting to the other store. If you can save money by going to two stores, then do it.

Watch those ad specials. Understand that the only reason they run specials is to get you into the store. The store will raise prices on items people purchase all the time to save money on the sale items. During the week before Thanksgiving last year, the store where we shop was running all kinds of specials. However, an item that we purchase about twice a month had been raised by five dollars!

Buy in bulk only if you use the item on a regular basis and only if you have adequate storage capacity, or if purchasing six of something is cheaper than purchasing four. You can always trade the other two items for something you want from a friend. Earlier, I mentioned that potatoes are cheaper by the bag; so are apples. If you purchase potatoes and a friend purchases apples, you can share. I met a woman who had this technique down to such a science that between coupons, sales, and purchasing in bulk, she was feeding a family of four on fifty dollars a week!

Become an expert at coupons, sales prices, purchasing in bulk, and food cooperative, and watch your food dollars go down. Remember, grocery stores are in business to make money—you have to play their game, but you can play to win!

Utilities

Gas, Electric, Water: You can save on these in a couple of ways. First, make sure your house or apartment is properly insulated. Most utility companies will come out and do an energy efficiency test and let you know how to save on your bill. Turn out the lights in rooms not being used. Keep the refrigerator door closed in hot weather. Don't leave the water running. Do full loads of laundry. Take a 5-10 minute shower instead of a bath. If you've got kids, wash several at once!

Some utility companies offer reduced monthly bills to folks with a limited income or senior citizens. Others will determine what your average monthly bill is and invoice that amount each month so it's easier to budget.

Clothes

Wow. I love clothes. I have sewn since I was nine years old. However, if you stop and think about it, clothes are expensive, they don't hold their value, and they go out of style within six months. The overriding truth, though, is that your clothes speak volumes about who you are. The good news is, you can look great, be in fashion, and do it economically.

However, most Americans go overboard when it comes to buying clothes. Here is an interesting thought from a British fellow I once worked with.

Dan moved his family, a wife and daughter, to Orlando, Florida from London, England. One day, he shook his head in disbelief. The day before, his wife had gone out and spent hundreds of dollars on clothes for the entire family. He said, "Jayne, my wife has decided she needs all those clothes like you Americans! Last night, I tried to explain it to her. You can only wear one thing at a time, so you buy two outfits, one to wear while the other one is washing. What is so complicated about that?"

Although two outfits isn't my idea of a wardrobe, he did make a lot of sense. We want to have the luxury of a clothing store in our closets so when we get dressed, we have choices. I am just as guilty as anyone else. I have clothes in my closet that still have the tags on them. My justification is that they were on sale. A $125 evening dress for $35 is a great deal! Not really; it's been in my closet now for two years and never been worn. Investing that money would have been a smarter idea. Buy only what you need right now. If and only if you have extra money should you buy ahead, because you can save money shopping out of season. For example, a black turtleneck sweater is a standard article of clothing in my closet. After five years, mine was getting ragged. So last spring, I purchased a black turtle neck sweater 75% off and wore it six months later.

Purchase colors that look good on you, especially for business wear. There are books you can borrow from the library about what colors work best for you. Learn what your core colors and accessories are. You will end up spending less money, and you will wear the clothes you do buy.

OK ladies, this one is going to freak you out! I own two pair of heels: black and navy blue. They go with every business outfit I own. I only carry a black purse or briefcase. There's no need for every color to match every outfit.

A well known celebrity said something years ago that has always stuck with me, and has saved me perhaps thousands of dollars: Buy black skirts or pants, wear black hose, and black shoes. Spend your money on tops. Most people don't look below your waistline anyway, and they'll always remember your blouse rather than your skirt. Plus, black has a slimming effect. Men's business outfits are pretty easy compared to women's: Black pants, solid or print shirt. I believe men who wear neckties enjoy expressing their personalities through them.

Children's Clothes

Children grow. That's what they are made to do — so you will be shopping a lot for them. If you follow the same principles for them as I've outlined for you, you will spend less. Here is one added ingredient: Only buy designer labels for special occasions. Advertisers have done a great job convincing us that our children need a $150 pair of shoes to feel good about themselves, when in fact it's the parent that feels good that his or her child is wearing a $150 pair of shoes. Get back to reality. What signal are you sending your children? That they can't feel good unless their shoes cost that kind of money?

If your kids are old enough, have them work and pay part of the cost. It will make them appreciate their clothes and treat them better.

When I didn't work, I washed clothes twice a week. The kids may have had three pairs of pants each at that time. When I went to work, I increased that to five pair, so I wouldn't have to do laundry in the middle of the week. They had two pairs of shoes, tennis shoes and church shoes. One sweater and one warm jacket were plenty.

As they moved into junior high, they wanted to buy their own clothes. I figured out a budget, and twice a year I took them shopping, always at sale time. I gave them each the same amount of money and sent them off into the stores to purchase what they wanted.

Each one came back with their arms full of clothes except one son. He came back with two items. He was the oldest one living at home and he wanted designer everything. I laughed and suggested he take them back so he could get what he really needed. No, he said, he wanted the designer labels. He was also working, so he ended up with two complete outfits to go with what he already had. He continued the tradition for five years. He wore the best designer clothes money could buy. Now, at 31 with a family of his own, he laughs at that stage in his life.

Shopping

If you are just getting into the business world and don't have a lot of money to spend on clothes, here are a couple of suggestions: contact your local Chamber of Commerce, shelters, or other help organizations, and see if they donate clothes for men and women who are trying to get back into the workforce. The Chamber I belong to does, and I recently donated three business suits.

Next, check with secondhand stores and consignment shops. Be careful, because some of these stores charge more than regular clothing stores. I have seen clothes sell for as much in these stores as in the regularly priced stores. If you can't get the item for 75% below the store's discount price, shop sales at regularly priced stores.

Sew if you have the time do it. Sewing has been both a blessing and a curse for me, because when I shop for clothes, I sometimes feel the quality of the items isn't worth the money. My friends and family will hear me say, "I could make that 80-90% cheaper." Now my problem is time. Sewing takes time and patience.

Buy clothes that fit. Don't buy clothes with the idea that you'll take up that hem or sew that seam unless you have the talent and time. If you do, then you can pick up some great deals. For me, sewing an entire outfit is easier than mending something.

High Priced Stores vs. Economy Priced Stores

Just the other day, I took my mother shopping at an economy store. We were trying to find her a long skirt when I noticed a blouse on a rack that looked familiar. I pulled it off the rack and, sure enough, this $14.95 blouse I was holding was exactly like the one I'd seen at a boutique for $75.

Buying clothes is an investment, not unlike years ago when people had one dress for church and a couple for every day. Make no mistake about it: clothes will tell people who you are, where you come from and your desire for the future.

Don't make the mistake that you <u>HAVE</u> to spend a lot of money on clothes to impress others. You can accomplish this by knowing quality, watching sales, and frequenting consignment shops and secondhand stores.

If you look at your business clothes as an investment, you should purchase high quality clothes that will last a long time. You should buy traditional clothes on which to build your wardrobe. Stay with neutral colors, and launder them properly. You will find that it all pays off in the long run. So if you invest $2,000 on a foundation wardrobe that will last two years, that breaks down to $1,000 a year, which is $83 per month, and only $21 a week. Use accessories to add variety and spice.

Here's a tip on clothes from a model and shop-aholic who is a friend of mine. Most of the money is made on the first ten items sold. The store hopes these first ten items will sell within the first two to three weeks. Then they start discounting, and continue to discount until they pull them off the racks. These items either go to the store's own factory outlet store or they sell them to another discount chain.

Just like at the grocery store, know what items are at the stores in your area. Learn the sales cycles for each store you shop in. Make a wardrobe list of what you have, what you need, and what you want. When someone asks you what you'd like for your birthday, you can pull out the list. You can even tell them where to get it! Most importantly, DON'T BUY ON IMPULSE! Remember, the first ten items sold are where the department stores make their profit.

Credit Cards

Don't use them if you can't pay the balance off each and every month for years. Do the math: if you save 10%

on your clothes but the credit card interest each month is 18%, did you really save money?

In order to succeed in money management, you need to be brutally honest. Every item on your expense list must be reviewed monthly. Remember, self-mastery is victory over a situation and leads to self-empowerment. Being honest with yourself as to what your wants and needs are will bring you that victory and move you closer to self-empowerment.

Knowledge Saves Money

Read labels and know what you are purchasing. Get to know the stores in your area. Consider mail orders. Purchases items your family always uses in bulk. Shop around for telephone long distance rates. Learn how to conserve energy. In other words, educate yourself in the art of frugality. Learn how pennies saved add up to dollars saved.

This lesson was a very expensive one for me to learn. Back in the '70s, I spent $7,000 on a solar unit to heat water. Boy, they saw us coming! AFTER the purchase, I determined that it would take 20 years to recover the cost. My marriage didn't even last that long. As it turned out, the unit was out of date, and broke within four years of its purchase; but we were still making monthly payments on it at the time of the divorce.

I wish I had just taken the time to educate myself about solar units. If I had figured out the cost over 20 years, and realized the return on my investment, I would have saved $7,000!

Save It

A savings account is for purchases in the future and/ or emergencies. Now that you have all of your income and expenses, record anything extra you should SAVE! Save every penny! You earned it; why not? Pennies add up to nickels, nickels add up to dimes, dimes to quarters, quarters to dollars, dollars to fives, fives to 10s to 20s to 100s — getting the picture? Case in point: you know five dollars goes faster than you can blink your eye. When I was 20 and pregnant with my second son, I found a way to put five dollars in a savings account from my paycheck each week.

A year later, I was able to purchase a solid oak dining table with that money. That's how fast it can add up. Build yourself a nest egg. What are you going to use your nest egg for? So many, many things like a car when yours breaks, a computer to help in your education, or a vacation.

Invest It

While a savings account is for your short-term purchase, an investment plan is for your retirement. If you haven't already started thinking about it, you should. Start now: reading, asking, and finding out what all the options are in the investing world.

You may never work for a company with a retirement program, so it could be up to you to plan for your own retirement. Think about this! Many seniors today are living on less than $900 per month, because the government told them and millions of other Americans back in the 1920s they would be taken care of with Social Security. No one knew what was really going to happen.

Plan your own future; don't let anyone else plan it for you.

Reality Check

If at this point you are frustrated with the fact that it is all up to you to earn money, save it, and spend it wisely, you're right! It is frustrating, and it *is* up to you. Let me share with you a little-known fact that I believe most Americans don't understand.

Advertising agencies get thousands and thousands of dollars to make you think that you will be prettier, smarter, more popular, sexier, and richer if you have their clients' products and services. They are good at what they do. They will use whatever means it takes to sell you on their clients' products: celebrities, athletes, or models. They are in the business to get you to buy whatever they are selling.

When I worked for the Cally Curtis Company, we were making training videos for business about time management, customer service, team building, etc. Cally used well known actors in her videos, so prospective clients would listen to what this actor had to say. It didn't matter that the actors didn't know a thing about customer service. People believed them because they saw them on television and at the movies.

Once you understand that these companies have been playing a game and that it's not necessarily for your benefit, it's up to you to figure out the game. If you play with the big boys, then play to win. Those guys want your money, whether you make ten million dollars a year or $10,000. They don't care about you; they want to win. Be a smart, informed shopper and you and your family will win.

Conclusion

Conclusion

Hopefully, the end of this book is the beginning of your new self-empowered life. There is no preconceived notion on my part that this has been a masterfully written book, but instead it has been a labor of love and devotion to Our Heavenly Father. For without Him being with me through my entire life on this earth I wouldn't be here to write these words.

From the moment the idea come to me to write this book seven years ago to the many rewrites and the typing of this page, the PURPOSE—the only purpose of this book—was to help one woman, one man, or one child to realize from my experiences, that you can, in fact, overcome unspeakable things that have happened to you and become the person you have only been dreaming about in secret. You can break a cycle of abuse in your family! You have the right to live your life as you choose, not one that was chosen for you. Every child has the right to live his or her life free of terror and pain.

Wherever you or I decide to go or whatever we decide to do from this moment forward doesn't really matter. What's important is that we do it with self-empowerment. I have learned to make my own decisions and learn from them, and you can, too. Lastly, don't ever forget what life is:

Life is Hard;
Get over It!

Life is an Adventure;
Explore It!

Life is Complicated;
Unravel It!

Life is Wonderful;
Enjoy It!

Life is Fearful;
Conquer It!

Life is a Puzzle;
Solve It!

Life is a Journey;
Travel It!

Life is to be Lived;
So Go Live It!

How "A Wallflower No More" Got Her Name

At the end of 1999, I found myself going through another divorce, this time with a different twist. The boys were on their own, so I was to be single without children. This newfound freedom felt awesome; for the first time in my life, I could do anything and go anywhere I wanted without consulting anyone.

New Year's Eve 2000 found me lying on a blanket in an empty apartment which was ready to be filled in a week. As I was ringing in the New Year by myself, enjoying this newly found solitude, my thoughts wandered over my life. At some point during the evening, I paused to consider my high school experiences. Not a pleasant memory. Then it dawned on me to exchange the negative memories with positive ones. As luck would have it, my 30 year high school reunion was the very next year, 2001. I started making plans to attend it.

On the day of the reunion, I was staying with my mother. She had gone to visit friends in Orange County, so I was left alone to get ready. All the depression of those unhappy school years came rushing in on me. I stood in the living room telling myself that I didn't need to go through this experience; after all, I was 48 years old, owned my own company, had just moved back to California, and was happy. Why go mess that up? So I sat down to watch television.

Just then the phone rang. It was my dear friend from Orlando, Florida. She suspected that I might back out and had called to wish me good luck. It took several minutes for her to realize I wasn't going, and as any good friend would, she said, "Get off your butt, get ready and go to that reunion." Special friends are just wonderful.

In 15 minutes I was headed for Loma Linda Country Club. As I was driving, I thought to myself that this would be a good time for the Los Angeles traffic to cause me to show up extremely late – say, at midnight. But of course the traffic on that Saturday evening in August was flowing freely, as if pushing me faster and faster toward this event in my life.

As I walked into the country club, I thought what a good time it would be for a late afternoon thunderstorm, so I would get soaked and would have a good excuse to go home. But of course I was in L.A., not Orlando, and there wasn't a cloud in the sky.

As I stood in line to register, I thought this would be a great time for a sudden attack of laryngitis – with my voice completely gone, I couldn't possibly carry on a conversation with anyone, and would be completely justified in going home early, like five minutes after my arrival. No such luck.

Instead, I struck up a conversation with the couple in front of me. The typical questions came up. What's your name? Who did you know in high school? Were you on any of the sports teams, or in any of the cool clubs? And for me, since I was standing by myself, are you married?

Quickly I realized I didn't know anyone, hadn't played on any sports teams or joined any cool clubs. I was totally out of my comfort zone. This feeling of being out of control became worse when another couple came up behind me and knew the couple in front of me. Suddenly, I was a fifth wheel, pushed aside as if I weren't there.

Instantly I was back in high school, with a pimply face, out-of-style clothes, and no makeup. I was a teenage nerd. I was frozen in time now, unable to speak when I finally got up to the registration table. I managed to croak out my name, but the woman behind the table didn't hear me and shouted, "What is your name?" I wanted to die on the spot. Finally she handed me my nametag; I was rushed off by another woman to wait in another line to have my picture taken. The photographer turned to me, looked around and asked, "Are you alone?"

All I could do was nod my head. Couldn't he see I was dying here? Why had I let Lisa talk me into coming to this event? My four years of high school were a nightmare; why was I putting myself through this again?

After the picture was taken, I walked down a little hallway. To my left was the designated ballroom – to my right, a bathroom. I sprinted to the safety of the bathroom – thank goodness it was empty – and jumped into a stall before anyone saw me. By this time, I was physically sick and just wanted to go home and spare myself any more pain. I didn't move; instead I concentrated on breathing and, as my mind cleared and I returned to being 48 instead of 18, I realized once again that the bastards had taken my childhood.

I practiced self-talk for 20 minutes in that stall as women came and went. As each minute passed, I became more self-empowered. After all, I was the woman who called Donald Trump's office to sell him videos; I was the woman who sold advertising to Bell South Mobility and the United States Post Office. I was the woman who had broken the cycle of abuse in my family. If I could do all that, then this little 30-year high school reunion would be a cakewalk.

Armed now with self-confidence and a plan, I walked out of that bathroom with my shoulders squared and my head held high. Walking into the ballroom, I stepped to my right as I was taught in etiquette class. Surveying the room, I saw several tables with people sitting at them talking away. To my right was the bar, so I slowly walked to the line, looking from side to side.

A man walked up behind me. My sales training on how to talk to anyone about anything kicked in, and I struck up a conversation with him. He introduced me to the man in front of me, who turned out to be our high school quarterback, now a successful doctor. The conversation came to the same questions as when I was registering. What clubs were you in? What sports did you play? My new plan kicked in; the moment of truth was at hand.

"Oh," I said, "you don't know me. I was one of the nerdy kids in high school, but that doesn't matter now, because I don't know you either." Both men started laughing. I was once again empowered, and the internal fear was gone.

After getting a tonic water with a twist of lime, I turned around to figure out where I was going to sit. To my surprise, the quarterback was waiting to escort me to his table, which turned out to be where the ex-cheerleaders and ex-football players were sitting. I had arrived!

However, I didn't stop there. After chatting to the people at the popular table, I decided to meet more of my fellow classmates. I went to all 10 tables, introducing myself this way: "Hi, I'm Jayne Maas (my maiden name). You don't know me, but that's okay because I don't know you, either."

What an icebreaker! Not only did it relax me, but the other people were also relaxing, making new friends, dancing, and totally enjoying themselves.

As the evening came to a close, the centerpieces were being raffled off. Engaged in a conversation (actually, landing a date) and not listening to what was going on, I suddenly heard my name being shouted by 30 people sitting at three different tables. I had won one of the door prizes. I felt like Cinderella at the ball!

That night, as I was driving home by myself, I suddenly thought to myself, "I am a wallflower no more!"

References

Books, music, movies, and yes, even TV, provided for me the "how to live life" knowledge I had missed while growing up. These sources guided me on how to start being a better mother, sister, daughter, and co-worker. My early social and interpersonal skills were learned though these mediums. Once I got myself to what I call a basic level, I took my education a step further; I started attending seminars on all types of topics. Grammar, learning personality types, interpersonal skills, how to talk to everyone, etiquette and leadership. I could gather the information, through one-day seminars, that I needed to continue my success; the time invested was minimal compared to what I got out of them. Usually, the company paid for the seminar; in addition to what the company paid, I have spent thousands of dollars on books, training videos, seminars, and audiotapes. But, you'd be amazed at what you can find in used bookstores or online for a fraction of the original price.

Biographies are a great place to start. It doesn't matter if you read about women or men, past or present. When you read about someone else's life, his or her struggles and triumphs, you realize you, too, can affect your own life, overcome struggles and get to where you want to go. Below are just a few of my favorites and the reasons why.

Eleanor Roosevelt – wife to Franklin, the President of the United States. She was the First Lady during the depression. Her famous quote is stated earlier in this book, "No one can make you feel inferior without your permission."

Cher – the singer. A few years after Sonny and Cher divorced, Cher wrote a book about her life before, during and after Sonny. She talked about how controlling and demanding Sonny was. Cher credited Sonny for being there when no one else was; he was determined to make their music a success, which gave her a foundation for the rest of her successful career. What I learned from Cher's book is that when someone is hard on you; maybe they see something in you that you don't see.

Georgia O'Keeffe – painter. Ms. O'Keeffe was a painter in the 1920s with many of her paintings being extremely controversial for her day. Many believed the flowers she painted were female sex organs. She never stopped painting what she wanted to paint, despite what others said. From her, I learned to trust myself.

Sharing the Wealth: My Story, Alex Spanos (Regnery Publishing, Inc., 2002) – Mr. Spanos has been a resident of Stockton, California his entire life. He went from working in his father's bakery to becoming a millionaire. He gives millions of dollars to the Stockton community. In recognition of his Greek heritage, President Bush asked him to represent the United States at the Olympic Games in Athens. Mr. Spanos is a great example of giving to the community which made him the man he is today.

Charlie's Monument, by Blaine M. Yorgason (Deseret Books, 2000) Although fiction, this book brings me to tears every time I read it. It's the story of a young man deformed at birth, and teased as a child and adult, who chose, in spite of his disabilities to become a vital part of his community. He plays the key role in saving this small western town from Indians. This book helped me realize I can do anything I want if I set my mind to the challenge.

Good-bye, I Love You, by Carol Lynn Pearson (Gold Leaf Press, 1997), is the true story of a wife, her homosexual husband and a love honored for time and all eternity. A powerful story of self-giving.

Tuesdays with Morrie, by Mitch Albom (Broadway, 2002). Mitch writes about the last weeks he spent with his mentor. What amazed me about this book is the love and compassion these two men have for each other.

If you don't know where to start reading, find someone you admire; most likely there will be a book written about him or her.

Business books and audiotapes will help you find a career, advance a career, or enhance a career. They certainly helped me find and advance my sales career. I also read many books about abuse, relationships, and living life that were invaluable to my success. Below is just a sampling of what is out there.

Araphakis, Maria. *How To Speak Up, Set Limits and Say No Without Losing Your Job or Your Friends.* Recording. CareerTrack Publications, 1986.

Bass, Ellen and Davis, Laura. *The Courage to Heal A Guide for Women Survivors of Child Sexual Abuse.* First ed. Harper-Collins Publishers, 1988.

Bayan, Richard. *Words That Sell.* Contemporary Books Inc., 1994.

Bolton & Bolton. *People Styles at Work: Making Bad Relationships Good and Good Relationships Better.* New York: AMACOM, a division of the American Management Association, 1996.

Buzan, Tony. *Make the Most of Your Mind.* New York: Linden Press/Simon and Schuster, 1984.

Carnegie, Dale. *How to Win Friends & Influence People.* Pocket Books, a division of Simon & Schuster, 1936.

Covey, Steven R. *Seven Habits of Highly Effective People.* Audiotape. Provo, Utah: Steven R. Covey & Associates, 1984.

Child Welfare Research Center. March 2005. U of Berkeley Center for Social Services Research. <http://cssr.berkeley.edu/childwelfare/>.

Deutsch, Georg and Sally P. Springer. *Left Brain, Right Brain.* W.H. Freeman & Company, 1998.

Fisher, Donna. *Power Networking.* Audiotape. CareerTrack.

Friedman, Dr. Sonya. *On a Clear Day You can See Yourself.* Ballantine Books, 1991.

Friedman, Nancy. *The Telephone Doctor.* Audiotape. St. Louis, MO: 1988.

Harvey, Ph.D., John R. *Total Relaxation.* Kodansha America, Inc., 1998.

Hill, Napoleon. *Think and Grow Rich*. New York: Fawcett Crest, 1960.

Johnson, M.D., Spencer. *Who Moved My Cheese?* G.P. Putnam's Sons, 1998.

Kroeger, Otto and Janet M. Thuesen. *Type Talk*. Dell Publishing, 1988.

LeBoueuf Ph.D., Michael. *How To Win Customers and Keep Them for Life*. New York: G.P. Putnam's Sons, 1987.

Loehr, James E. *Stress for Success*. Times Books, a division of Random House, 1997.

MacKay, Harvey. *Beware The Naked Man Who Offers You His Shirt*. Ballantine Books, 1990.

MacKay, Harvey. *Swim With The Sharks Without Being Eaten Alive*. Ballantine Books, 1998.

---. *What They Don't Teach You at Harvard Business School*. Bantam Books, 1984.

McCutcheon, Marc. *The Compass in Your Nose and Other Astonishing Facts About Humans*. Jeremy P. Tarcher/Putnam, 1989.

Miller, Debra Sands. *Independent Women: Creating Our Lives, Living Our Visions*. Wildcat Canyon Press, a division of Circulus Publishing Group, 1998.

National Clearinghouse on Child Abuse and Neglect. March 2005., <http://nccanch.acf.hhs.gov>

Nelson, Bob. *1001 Ways to Energize Employees*. Workman Publishing, 1997.

---. *1001 Ways to Reward Employees*. Workman Publishing, 1994.

Olsen, David. *The Words You Should Know: 1200 Essential Words Every Educated Person Should be Able to Use and Define*. Bob Adams Inc., 1991.

Peck, M.D., M. Scott. *The Road Less Traveled*. Simon & Schuster, 1978.

Peter, Thomas J. and Robert H. Waterman, Jr. *In Search of Excellence*. Warner Books Edition, 1982.

Pinskey, Raleigh. *101 Ways to Promote Yourself*. Avon Books, 1997.

Robbins, Anthony. *Notes from a Friend*. Simon & Schuster, 1991.

Rovaris-MacDonald, Pearl. Audiotape. *How to Think Creatively*. SkillPath Publications, 1998.

Shear, Barbara. *I Could Do Anything, If I Only Knew What It Was*. Dell Publishing, 1994.

Stanley, Ph.D., Thomas J. and William D. Danko, Ph.D. *The Millionaire Next Door*. Pocket Books, a division of Simon & Schuster, 1996.

Tracy, Brian. Audiotape. *The Psychology of Selling, The Art of Closing Sales*. Nightingale Conant.

Ward, Francine. *Esteemable Acts*. New York: Random House, Inc., 2003.

Ziegler, Ph.D., Dave. *Raising Children Who Refuse To Be Raised*. Phoenix, AZ: Acacia Publishing, 2000.

Ziegler, Ph.D., Dave. *Traumatic Experience and The Brain.* Phoenix, AZ: Acacia Publishing, 2002.

Power and Control Wheel

Physical and sexual assaults, or threats to commit them, are the most apparent forms of domestic violence and are usually the actions that allow others to become aware of the problem. However, regular use of other abusive behaviors by the batterer, when reinforced by one or more acts of physical violence, make up a larger system of abuse. Although physical assaults may occur only once or occasionally, they instill threat of future violent attacks and allow the abuser to take control of the woman's life and circumstances.

The Power & Control diagram is a particularly helpful tool in understanding the overall pattern of abusive and violent behaviors, which are used by a batterer to establish and maintain control over his partner. Very often, one or more violent incidents are accompanied by an array of these other types of abuse. They are less easily identified, yet firmly establish a pattern of intimidation and control in the relationship.

Power and Control Diagram

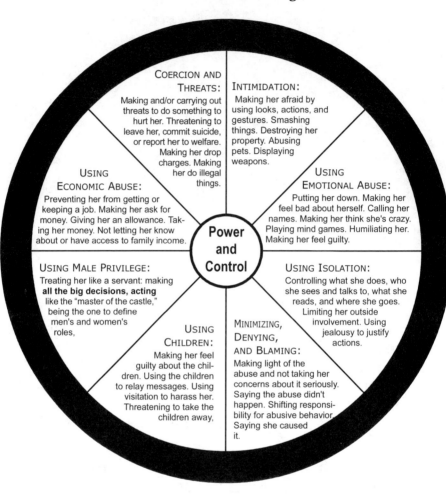

COERCION AND THREATS:
Making and/or carrying out threats to do something to hurt her. Threatening to leave her, commit suicide, or report her to welfare. Making her drop charges. Making her do illegal things.

INTIMIDATION:
Making her afraid by using looks, actions, and gestures. Smashing things. Destroying her property. Abusing pets. Displaying weapons.

USING ECONOMIC ABUSE:
Preventing her from getting or keeping a job. Making her ask for money. Giving her an allowance. Taking her money. Not letting her know about or have access to family income.

USING EMOTIONAL ABUSE:
Putting her down. Making her feel bad about herself. Calling her names. Making her think she's crazy. Playing mind games. Humiliating her. Making her feel guilty.

Power and Control

USING MALE PRIVILEGE:
Treating her like a servant: making **all the big decisions, acting** like the "master of the castle," being the one to define men's and women's roles,

USING ISOLATION:
Controlling what she does, who she sees and talks to, what she reads, and where she goes. Limiting her outside involvement. Using jealousy to justify actions.

USING CHILDREN:
Making her feel guilty about the children. Using the children to relay messages. Using visitation to harass her. Threatening to take the children away,

MINIMIZING, DENYING, AND BLAMING:
Making light of the abuse and not taking her concerns about it seriously. Saying the abuse didn't happen. Shifting responsibility for abusive behavior. Saying she caused it.

Power and Control Wheel courtesy of:
Domestic Abuse Intervention Project
202 East Superior Street
Duluth, Minnesota 55802
218-722-2781

Resources

National Organizations with Local Chapters

The following national organizations and programs have local chapters in States and communities across the country. Please call the national office or go to the Web site listing to identify a local office near you.

Alliance for Children and Families

The Alliance for Children and Families, an international membership association, represents more than 350 private, nonprofit child- and family-serving organizations providing a vast array of services ranging from residential care to abuse prevention and intervention.
Phone: (414) 359-1040
Web site: www.alliance1.org

AVANCE Family Support and Education Program

AVANCE provides support and education services to low-income families to strengthen their family, enhance parenting skills to nurture the optimal development of children, promote educational success, and foster the personal and economic success of parents.
Phone: (210) 270-4630
Web site: www.avance.org
Local contacts: www.avance.org (See link for "Contact.")

Healthy Families America®

Healthy Families America®, a program of Prevent Child Abuse America, promotes positive parenting and child health and development through voluntary home visits by trained staff.

Phone: (312) 663-3520
Web site: www.healthyfamiliesamerica.org
Local contacts: www.healthyfamiliesamerica.org/state_system_locator/index.shtml

Meld

Meld offers educational and support services for parents, trains family service providers to apply best practices, and publishes resource materials for parents and service providers.

Phone: (612) 332-7563
Web site: www.meld.org
Local contacts: www.meld.org/sitemaplist.cfm

Child Welfare League of America (CWLA)

CWLA is an association of more than 1,100 public and private nonprofit agencies that coordinate national and local child abuse prevention efforts and assist over 3.5 million abused and neglected children and their families each year with a wide range of services.

Phone: (202) 638-2954
Web site: www.cwla.org
Local contacts: www.cwla.org/members/members.htm

Circle of Parents™

Circle of Parents™ is a national network of organizations that provide parent self-help support groups to anyone in a parenting role. These groups offer parents a place to discuss the challenges of raising kids, exchange ideas, and offer support. Circle of Parents™ is a collaborative project of Prevent Child Abuse America and the National Family Support Roundtable, and is sponsored by OCAN and OJJDP.

Phone: (312) 663-3520
Web site: www.circleofparents.org
Local contacts: www.circleofparents.org/locator/index.html

Family Support America (FSA)

Family Support America promotes family support for ensuring the well-being of our children. FSA advocates on behalf of families and provides technical assistance, training and education, conferences, and publications.

Phone: (312) 338-0900
Web site: www.familysupportamerica.org
Local contacts: www.familysupportamerica.org/content/mapping_dir/find.asp

FRIENDS (Family Resource Information, Education and Network Services) National Resource Center for Community-Based Grants for the Prevention of Child Abuse and Neglect

FRIENDS provides technical assistance and information to State leads of Community-Based Grants for the Prevention of Child Abuse and Neglect to help States in their efforts of reducing the incidence of child abuse and neglect and strengthening families.

Phone: (312) 338-0900
Web site: www.friendsnrc.org
Local contacts: www.friendsnrc.org

The National Alliance of Children's Trust and Prevention Funds

The National Alliance of Children's Trust and Prevention Funds initiates and engages in national efforts that assist State Children's Trust and Prevention Funds in strengthening families to prevent child abuse and neglect. Children's Trust and Prevention Funds annually provide more than $100 million for community-based child abuse and neglect prevention programs that serve 2 million families.

Phone: (517) 432-5096

Web site: www.ctfalliance.org

Local contacts: www.ctfalliance.org (See link for "Participating States.")

National Exchange Club Foundation for the Prevention of Child Abuse (NECF)

The NECF coordinates a nationwide network of community-based Exchange Club Child Abuse Prevention Centers, which offer a professionally supervised parent aide program—based on Erikson's stages of development—to at-risk parents, with the goal of replacing traditional patterns of abusive behavior with effective skills for nonviolent parenting.

Phone: (800) 924-2643

Web site: www.preventchildabuse.com

Local contacts: www.preventchildabuse.com/usamap.htm

Parents Anonymous® Inc.

Parents Anonymous® Inc. leads a dynamic international network of accredited organizations that implement weekly, ongoing Parents Anonymous® Adult and Children's Groups that are free of charge to participants and based on a shared leadership model.

Phone: (909) 621-6184

Web site: www.parentsanonymous.org

Prevent Child Abuse America

With chapters in nearly 40 States and the District of Columbia Prevent Child Abuse America provides leadership to promote and implement child abuse prevention efforts at both the national and local levels.

Phone: (312) 663-3520

Web site: www.preventchildabuse.org

Local contacts: www.preventchildabuse.org/get local/ index.html

National Organizations that Provide Information, Training, and Technical Assistance

The following national organizations are among many that provide information and services to support the prevention of child abuse and neglect. Inclusion on this list is for information purposes and does not constitute an endorsement.

American Professional Society on the Abuse of Children (APSAC)

The American Professional Society on the Abuse of Children is a national, multidisciplinary organization that works to improve the practice of professionals in the field of child abuse and neglect. Phone: (405) 271-8202

Web site: www.apsac.org

ARCH National Respite Network and Resource Center

The ARCH National Respite Network and Resource Center promotes the development of respite and crisis care programs, helps families locate respite and crisis care, and serves as a voice for respite in all forums.

Phone: (800) 473-1727, Ext. 222

Web site: www.archrespite.org/ARCHserv.htm

Childhelp USA®

In addition to a 24-hour National Child Abuse Hotline (1-800-4-A-CHILD®), Childhelp USA® directly serves abused children through residential treatment facilities, child advocacy centers, group homes, foster care, preschool programs (including Head Start), child abuse prevention programs, and community outreach.
Phone: (480) 922-8212
Web site: www.childhelpusa.org

Children's Defense Fund

The Children's Defense Fund focuses on key issues affecting the well-being of children by helping develop, implement, and monitor State and Federal policies.
Phone: (202) 628-8787
Web site: www.childrensdefense.org

Coalition for Marriage, Family and Couples Education (CMFCE)

CMFCE serves as a clearinghouse to help people find the information they need to strengthen marriages — their own or those in their community. CMFCE connects those with an interest in the ongoing development of marriage and family education; promotes awareness of the effectiveness of the educational approach; and works to increase the availability and quality of courses and programs in the community.
Phone: (202) 362-3332
Web site: www.smartmarriages.com

International Society for the Prevention of Child Abuse and Neglect (ISPCAN)

ISPCAN, a member society with benefits including *Child Abuse and Neglect: The International Journal*, brings together a worldwide cross-section of professionals to work toward the prevention of child abuse and neglect, and exploitation globally by increasing public awareness, developing activities to prevent violence, and promoting the rights of children all over the world.
Phone: (630) 221-1311
Web site: www.ispcan.org

Kempe Children's Center

The Kempe Children's Center provides clinical treatment, training, research, education, and program development to prevent and treat child abuse and neglect.
Phone: (303) 864-5252
Web site: www.kempecenter.com

National Clearinghouse on Child Abuse and Neglect Information

The Clearinghouse provides information products and technical assistance services to help professionals locate information related to child abuse and neglect and related child welfare issues.
Phone: (800) 394-3366
Web site: http://nccanch.acf.hhs.gov

National Council on Child Abuse and Family Violence (NCCAFV)

NCCAFV works to strengthen community child abuse and family violence prevention and treatment programs across the country through public awareness and education, professional development, and organizational development.
Phone: (202) 429-6695
Web site: http://nccafv.org

National Indian Child Welfare Association (NICWA)

NICWA is a membership organization of Tribes, individuals, and private organizations that works to promote Indian child welfare and address child abuse and neglect through training, research, public policy, and grassroots community development.

Phone: (503) 222-4044

Web site: www.nicwa.org

Shaken Baby Syndrome Prevention Plus

Shaken Baby Syndrome Prevention Plus develops, studies, and disseminates information and materials designed to prevent Shaken Baby Syndrome and other forms of physical child abuse.

Phone: (800) 858-5222

Web site: www.sbsplus.com

Stop It Now!

Stop It Now! is a national nonprofit working to prevent and ultimately eradicate child sexual abuse. Stop It Now! challenges adults to take action by calling on abusers, adults at risk to abuse, and their friends and family, to come forward, learn the warning signs, and seek help. Using the tools of public health, Stop It Now! works to prevent child sexual abuse *before* it is perpetrated.

Phone: (413) 268-3096

Web site: www.stopitnow.org

Toll-Free Crisis Hotline Numbers

Childhelp USA

Phone: 800-4-A-CHILD (800-422-4453)

Who They Help: Child abuse victims, parents, concerned individuals

Youth Crisis Hotline

Phone: 800-HIT-HOME (800-448-4663)
Who They Help: Individuals reporting child abuse, youth ages 12 to 18

Stop It Now!

Phone: 888-PREVENT (888-773-8368)
Who They Help: Child sexual abuse victims, parents, offenders, concerned individuals

National Domestic Violence Hotline Phone: 800-799-SAFE (800-799-7233)

Who They Help: Children, parents, friends, offenders

Child Find of America

Phone: 800-1-AM-LOST (800-426-5678)
Who They Help: Parents reporting lost or abducted children

Child Find of America — Mediation

Phone: 800-A-WAY-OUT (800-292-9688)
Who They Help: Parents (abduction, prevention, child custody issues)

Child Quest International Sighting Line

Phone: 888-818-HOPE (888-818-4673)
Who They Help: Individuals with missing child emergencies and/or sighting information; victims of abduction

National Center for Missing and Exploited Children Phone: 800-THE-LOST (800-843-5678)

Who They Help: Families and professionals (social services, law enforcement)

Operation Lookout National Center for Missing Youth Phone: 800-LOOKOUT (800-566-5688)

Who They Help: Individuals with missing child emergencies and/or sighting information (for children ages 18 and under)

Rape and Incest National Network

Phone: 800-656-HOPE; Ext. 1 (800-656-4673; Ext. 1)

Who They Help: Rape and incest victims, media, policy makers, concerned individuals

National Respite Locator Service

Phone: 800-677-1116

Who They Help: Parents, caregivers, and professionals caring for children and adults with disabilities, terminal illnesses, or those at risk of abuse or neglect

Girls and Boys Town

Phone: 800-448-3000

Who They Help: Abused, abandoned, and neglected girls and boys; parents; family members

Covenant House Hotline

Phone: 800-999-9999

Who They Help: Problem teens and homeless runaways (ages 21 and under), family members, youth substance abusers

National Referral Network for Kids in Crisis

Phone: 800-KID-SAVE (800-543-7283)

Who They Help: Professionals, parents, adolescents

National Runaway Switchboard Phone: 800-621-4000

Who They Help: Runaway and homeless youth, families

National Youth Crisis Hotline (Youth Development International) Phone: 800-HIT-HOME (800-448-4663)

Who They Help: Individuals wishing to obtain help for runaways; youth (ages 12 to 18) experiencing drug abuse, teen pregnancy, homelessness, prostitution, or physical, emotional, or sexual abuse

Crime Victims

National Center for Victims of Crime

Phone: 800-FYI-CALL (800-394-2255)
Who They Help: Families, communities, and individuals harmed by crime

Other U.S. Organizations

The Center for Mental Health Services' Knowledge Exchange Network (KEN)

(English, Spanish). An award-winning government Web site that offers a wealth of information about mental health. Visitors can order free publications online, search KEN's referral database, read the latest mental health news, and explore links on a variety of mental health-related topics including child abuse, violence, depression, anxiety, substance abuse, self-help/support groups, treatment, and research.

Center for the Prevention of Sexual and Domestic Violence

936 N 34th Street, Suite 200,
Seattle, WA 98103
206-634-1903
fax 206-6340115

Children's Defense Fund

25 E Street
NW Washington, DC 20001
202-628-8787
Corporate Alliance to End Partner Violence
A national nonprofit organization working to prevent domestic violence. Founded by business leaders and focused on the workplace, its membership is comprised of US corporations and businesses united to educate and aid in the prevention of partner violence.

National Council on Child Abuse & Family Violence

1155 Connecticut Avenue, NW Suite 400
Washington, DC 20036
(202) 4296695 or (800) 222-2000

National Helpline National Committee for the Prevention of Elder Abuse c/o Institute on Aging Medical Center of Central Massachusetts

119 Belmont Street
Worcester, MA 01605
508-793-6166

National AIDS Network

P.O. Box 13827
Research Triangle Park, NC 27709
National AIDS Hotline 800-342-2437
TTY - 800-243-7889
Spanish - 800-344-7432

National Abortion and Reproductive Rights Action League

1156 15th Street, NW #700
Washington, DC 20005
202-973-3000
202-9733096-FAX

WHISPER (Women Hurt in Systems of Prostitution Engaged in Revolt)

P.O. Box 56796
St. Paul, MN 55165
612-644-6301

National Women's Political Caucus

1275 K Street, NW, Suite 750
Washington, DC 20005-4051

National Resource Center on Domestic Violence; Pennsylvania Coalition Against Domestic Violence

6400 Flank Drive, Suite 1300
Harrisburg, PA 17112
800-537-2238
717-5459456-FAX

Battered Women's Justice Project Minnesota Program Development, Inc.

http://www.ncadv.org/resources/other.htm
206 West Fourth Street
Duluth, MN 55806
800-903-0111
218-722-1545-FAX

Health Resource Center on Domestic Violence; Family Violence Prevention Fund

383 Rhode Island Street, Suite 304
San Francisco, CA 94103-5133
800-3131310
415-252-8991-FAX

Resource Center on Child Custody and Child Protection; National Council on Juvenile and Family Court Judges

P.O. Box 8970
Reno, NV 98507
800-527-3223
702-784-6628-FAX

National Coalition for Low-Income Housing

1012 14th Street, NW Suite 1200
Washington, DC 20005
202-662-1530

National Clearinghouse for the Defense of Battered Women

125 South 9th Street, Suite 302
Philadelphia, PA 19107
215-351-0010
215-357-0779-FAX
http://www.ncadv.org/resources/other.htm

California County Child Welfare Services Addresses and Reporting Telephone Numbers

ALAMEDA

Director, Alameda County CWS Agency
P.O. Box 12941
Oakland, CA 94607 510-259-1800

ALPINE

Director, Alpine County CWS Agency
75-A Diamond Valley Road
Markleeville, CA 96120
888-755-8099
24 hours 530-694-2235

AMADOR

Director, Amador County CWS Agency
1003 Broadway
Jackson, CA 95642
209-223-6550 days
209-223-1075 after hours

BUTTE

Director, Butte County CWS Agency
P.O. Box 1649
Oroville, CA 95965
530-538-7617 Oroville
800-400-0902 others

CALAVERAS

Director, Calaveras County CWS Agency
891 Mountain Ranch Road
San Andreas, CA 95249-9709
209-754-6452 days
209-754-6500 after hours

COLUSA

Director, Colusa County CWS Agency
P.O. Box 370
Colusa, CA 95932
530-458-0280

CONTRA COSTA

Director, Contra Costa County CWS Agency
40 Douglas Drive
Martinez, CA 94553-4068
925-646-1680 central
510-374-3324 west
510-925-427-8811 east

DEL NORTE

Director, Del Norte County CWS Agency
880 Northcrest Drive
Crescent City, CA 95531
707-464-3191

EL DORADO

Director, El Dorado County CWS Agency
3057 Briw Road
Placerville, CA 95667
530-544-7236 S. Tahoe
530-642-7100 Placerville

FRESNO

Director, Fresno County CWS Agency
2600 Ventura Street
Fresno, CA 93750
559-255-8320

GLENN

Director, Glenn County CWS Agency
P.O. Box 611
Willows, CA 95988
530-934-6520

HUMBOLDT

Director, Humboldt County CWS Agency
929 Koster Street
Eureka, CA 95501
707-445-6180

IMPERIAL

Director, Imperial County CWS Agency
2995 South 4th Street, Suite 105
El Centro, CA 92243
760-337-7750

INYO

Director, Inyo County CWS Agency
Courthouse Annex, Drawer A
Independence, CA 93526-0601
760-872-1727

KERN

Director, Kern County CWS Agency
PO Box 511
Bakersfield, CA 93302
661-631-6011 days

KINGS

Director, Kings County CWS Agency
1200 South Drive
Hanford, CA 93230
559-582-8776

LAKE

Director, Lake County CWS Agency
P.O. Box 9000
Lower Lake, California 95457
707-262-0235

LASSEN

Director, Lassen County CWS Agency
Post Office Box 1359
Susanville, CA 96130
530-251-8277 days
530-257-6121 Sheriff (after hours)

LOS ANGELES

Director, Los Angeles County CWS Agency
425 Shatto Place
Los Angeles, CA 90020
800-540-4000 In-State
213-639-4500 Out of State

MADERA

Director, Madera County CWS Agency
700 East Yosemite Avenue
Madera, CA 93638
559-675-7829
800-801-3999

MARIN

Director, Marin County CWS Agency
20 North San Pedro Rd, Suite 2028
San Rafael, CA 94903
415-499-7153
415-479-1601 TDD

MARIPOSA

Director, Mariposa County CWS Agency
5186 Highway 49
North Mariposa, CA 95338
209-966-3030

MENDOCINO

Director, Mendocino County CWS Agency
P.O. Box 1060
Ukiah, CA 95482
707-463-5600

MERCED

Director, Merced County CWS Agency
Post Office Box 112
Merced, CA 95341
209-385-3104 days
209-385 9915 (after hours)

MODOC

Director, Modoc County CWS Agency
120 North Main Street
Alturas, CA 96101
530-233-6501 days
530-233-4416 after hours

MONO

Director, Mono County CWS Agency
Post Office Box 576
Bridgeport, CA 93517
760-932-7755 or
800-340-5411 (statewide)

MONTEREY

Director, Monterey County CWS Agency
1000 South Main Street, Suite 209-A
Salinas, CA 93901
831-755-4661

NAPA

Director, Napa County CWS Agency
2261 Elm Street
Napa, CA 94559
707-253-4261

NEVADA

Director, Nevada County CWS Agency
P.O. Box 1210
Nevada City, CA 95959
530-265-9380

ORANGE

Director, Orange County CWS Agency
888 North Main Street
Santa Ana, CA 92701
714-940-1000
800-207-4464

PLACER

Director, Placer County CWS Agency
11730 Enterprise Drive
Auburn, CA 95603
530-886-5401
916-787-8860 Roseville/Rocklin/Granite Bay

PLUMAS

Director, Plumas County CWS Agency
270 County Hospital Road, Suite 207
Quincy, CA 95971
530-283-6350

RIVERSIDE

Director, Riverside County CWS Agency
4060 County Circle Drive
Riverside, CA 92503
800-442-4918

SACRAMENTO

Director, Sacramento County CWS Agency
7001 East Parkway, Suite A
Sacramento, CA 95823
916-875-5437

SAN BENITO

Director, San Benito County CWS Agency
1111 San Felipe Road, Suite 206
Hollister, CA 95023
831-636-4190 days
831-636-4330 after hours

SAN BERNARDINO

Director, San Bernardino County CWS Agency
385 North Arrowhead Avenue, 5th Floor
San Bernardino, CA 92415
800-827-8724
909-422-3266 after hours

SAN DIEGO
Director, San Diego County CWS Agency
1700 Pacific Highway, M.S. P501
San Diego, CA 92101
858-560-2191

SAN FRANCISCO
Director, San Francisco County CWS Agency
P. O. Box 7988
San Francisco, CA 94120
415-558-2650
800-856-5553

SAN JOAQUIN
Director, San Joaquin County CWS Agency
P.O. Box 201056
Stockton, CA 95201-3006
209-468-1333
209-468-1330

SAN LUIS OBISPO
Director, San Luis Obispo County CWS Agency
P. O. Box 8119
San Luis Obispo, CA 93403-8119
805-781-5437
800-834-5437

SAN MATEO
Director, San Mateo County CWS Agency
400 Harbor Blvd.
Belmont, CA 94002
650-595-7922
800-632-4615
650-595-7518 fax

SANTA BARBARA

Director, Santa Barbara County CWS Agency
234 Camino Del Remedio
Santa Barbara, CA 93110
800-367-0166 days
805-737-7078 Lompoc
805-683-2724 after hours

SANTA CLARA

Director, Santa Clara County CWS Agency
1725 Technology Drive
San Jose, CA 95110
408-299-2071 North
408-683-0601 South

SANTA CRUZ

Director, Santa Cruz County CWS Agency
1000 Emeline Avenue
Santa Cruz, CA 95060
831-454-4222
831-763-8850 Watsonville

SHASTA

Director, Shasta County CWS Agency
P.O. Box 496005
Redding, CA 96049-6005
530-225-5144

SIERRA

Director, Sierra County CWS Agency
P. O. Box 1019
Loyalton, CA 90118
530-289-3720 24 hours
530-993-6720 business hours only

SISKIYOU

Director, Siskiyou County CWS Agency
818 South Main Street
Yreka, CA 96097
530-841-4200 business hours only
530-842-7009 24 hours

SOLANO

Director, Solano County CWS Agency
P.O. Box 4090 MS 3-220
Fairfield, CA 94533
800-544-8696

SONOMA

Director, Sonoma County CWS Agency
P. 0. Box 1539
Santa Rosa, CA 95402-1539
707-565-4304

STANISLAUS

Director, Stanislaus County CWS Agency
P. O. Box 42
Modesto, CA 95353-0042
800-558-3665

SUTTER

Director, Sutter County CWS Agency
P. O. Box 1535
Yuba City, CA 95992-1535
530-822-7155

TEHAMA

Director, Tehama County CWS Agency
P.O. Box 1515
Red Bluff, CA 96080
800-323-7711
530-527-9416

TRINITY

Director, Trinity County CWS Agency
P. O. Box 1470
Weaverville, CA 96093-1470
530-623-1314

TULARE

Director, Tulare County CWS Agency
5957 South. Mooney Blvd
Visalia, CA 93277
800-331-1585 co. only
559-730-2677

TUOLUMNE

Director, Tuolumne County CWS Agency
20075 Cedar Road North
Sonora, CA 95370
209-533-5717 days
209-533-4357 after hours

VENTURA

Director, Ventura County CWS Agency
505 Poli Street
Ventura, CA 93001
805-654-3200

YOLO

Director, Yolo County CWS Agency
25 North Cottenwood Street
Woodland, CA 95695
530-669-2345
530 669-2346
530-666-8920 after hours
888-400-0022

YUBA

Director, Yuba County CWS Agency
P. O. Box 2320
Marysville, CA 95901
530-749-6288

Web Sites

Family Violence Prevention Fund
http://fvpf.org/

National Coalition Against Domestic Violence
http://www.ncadv.org

National Network to End Domestic Violence
http://www.nnedv.org

National Resource Center (NRC), a project of the Pennsylvania Coalition Against Domestic Violence
(800) 537-2238
http://www.pcadv.org

National Organization for Women
http://63.111.42.146/home/default.asp

Violence Against Women Office
http://www.ojp.usdoj.gov/vawo/

Women Matter
http://www.womenmatter.com/index.shtml

State Coalition List

To get help or give help call your State Coalition Office to rind the program offering shelter and support nearest to you:
- Alabama Coalition Against Domestic Violence
(334) 832-4842
- Alaska Network on Domestic Violence & Sexual Assault
(907) 586-3650
- Arizona Coalition Against Domestic Violence
(602) 279-2900
- Arkansas Coalition Against Domestic Violence
(800) 269-4668
- California Alliance Against Domestic Violence
(916) 444-7163
- Statewide California Coalition for Battered Women
(888) 722-2952
- Colorado Coalition Against Domestic Violence
(303) 831-9632
- Connecticut Coalition Against Domestic Violence
(860) 282-7899
- Delaware Coalition Against Domestic Violence
(302) 658-2958
- DC Coalition Against Domestic Violence
(202) 299-1181
- Florida Coalition Against Domestic Violence
(850 425-2749
- Georgia Coalition Against Domestic Violence
(404) 209-0280
- Hawaii State Coalition Against Domestic Violence
(808) 832-9316
- Idaho Coalition Against Sexual and Domestic Violence
(208) 384-0419
- Illinois Coalition Against Domestic Violence
(217) 789-2830
- Indiana Coalition Against Domestic Violence
(317) 917-3685
- Iowa Coalition Against Domestic Violence

(515) 244-8028
- Kansas Coalition Against Sexual & Domestic Violence
(785) 232-9784
- Kentucky Domestic Violence Association
(502) 695-2444
- Louisiana Coalition Against Domestic Violence
(504) 752-1296
- Maine Coalition for Family Crisis Services
(207) 941-1194
- Maryland Network Against Domestic Violence
(301) 352-4574
- Jane Doe, Inc./MA Coalition Against Sexual & Domestic Violence
(617) 248-0922
- Michigan Coalition Against Domestic Violence
(517) 347-7000
- Minnesota Coalition for Battered Women
(651) 646-6177
- Mississippi Coalition Against Domestic Violence
(601) 981-9196
- Missouri Coalition Against Domestic Violence
(573) 634-4161
- Montana Coalition Against Domestic Violence
(406) 443-7794
- Nebraska Domestic Violence and Sexual Assault Coalition
(402) 4766256
- Nevada Network Against Domestic Violence
(775) 828-1115
- New Hampshire Coalition Against Domestic & Sexual Violence
(603) 2248893
- New Jersey Coalition for Battered Women
(609) 584-8107
- New Mexico State Coalition Against Domestic Violence
(505) 246-9240
- New York State Coalition Against Domestic Violence
(518) 482-5465
- North Carolina Coalition Against Domestic Violence

(919) 956-9124
- North Dakota Council on Abused Women's Services
(701) 255-6240
- Ohio Domestic Violence Network
(614) 781-9651
- Action Ohio Coalition for Battered Women
(614) 221-1255
- Oklahoma Coalition on Domestic Violence and Sexual Assault
(405) 8481815
- Oregon Coalition Against Domestic and Sexual Violence
(503) 365-9644
- Pennsylvania Coalition Against Domestic Violence
(717) 545-6400
- Comision Para Los Asuntos De La Mujer, Puerto Rico
(787) 721-7676
- Rhode Island Council on Domestic Violence
(401) 467-9940
- South Carolina Coalition Against Domestic Violence & Sexual Assault
(803) 256-2900
- South Dakota Coalition Against Domestic Violence & Sexual Assault
(605) 945-0869
- Tennessee Task Force Against Family Violence
(615) 386-9406
- Texas Council on Family Violence
(512) 794-1133
- Utah Domestic Violence Advisory Council
(801) 538-4635
- Vermont Network Against Domestic Violence & Sexual Assault
(802) 2231302
- Virginians Against Domestic Violence
(757) 221-0990
- Washington State Coalition Against Domestic Violence
(360) 586-1022
- West Virginia Coalition Against Domestic Violence

(304) 965-3552
•Wisconsin Coalition Against Domestic Violence
(608) 255-0539
•Wyoming Coalition Against Domestic Violence &
Sexual Assault
(307) 7555481
•Women's Resource Center, Virgin Islands
(809) 776-3966
•Women's Coalition of St. Croix, Virgin Islands
(340) 773-9272